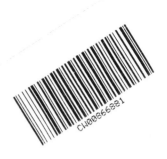

Healing Begins in the Kitchen

Louise

Use this for your

Very Best Health & to Enjoy

Cooking & eating again.

Enjoy

Be healthy!

Dr R. Minn

To Your
Abundant
Health ♡

Beth
Minn

Healing Begins in the Kitchen

Get Well and Stay There with the Misner Plan

Ivan Misner PhD
Beth Misner
Eddie Esposito
with Miguel Espinoza MD

ISBN: 1514228920
ISBN-13: 9781514228920
Library of Congress Control Number: 2015909217
CreateSpace Independent Publishing Platform
North Charleston, South Carolina

Dedication

We dedicate this book to our loved ones whom we have lost to cancer and other preventable diseases. If we can help even one person make the changes that will result in a long, healthy, and productive life, then our experiences with cancer will not have been in vain.

Beth and Ivan Misner: We would both like to dedicate this book to Jerry Ruth Misner, Ivan's mother. Mom was one of the most positive people we have both known. She struggled with her health for more than fifty years, including heart issues and cancer. Even in the face of serious health issues, she was cheerful and positive. We love you, Mom, and we miss you every day. Thank you for your inspiration in the face of so much difficulty.

Chef Eddie Esposito: I want to dedicate this book to my beautiful wife, Heather, and my three adored children, Jorden, Mattie, and Amelia, who make my life so rewarding and fulfilled. And to my father, Louis Esposito, who might have had a different outcome from the prostate cancer that took him too young if he'd had the Misner Plan available to him. My hope is that all our children will now benefit from this knowledge and live healthy, long, and productive lives.

Endorsements for *Healing Begins in the Kitchen*

"My wife, Tana, and I value greatly the importance of a healthy diet for a healthy life and brain. The Misners have made amazing changes in their eating habits and lifestyle, and the results speak for themselves. We know you will benefit from their experience and cannot encourage you more strongly to read their story."

—Dr. Daniel G. Amen and Tana Amen, coauthors of *The Brain Warrior's Way: Ignite Focus and Energy, Attack Illness and Aging, Turn Pain into Purpose*

"Ivan and Beth have done so much to educate themselves on how to eat to beat cancer. And they are sharing everything they have learned with us in this engaging book. Seeing how they allowed this experience to draw them closer together has been moving."

—Dr. John Gray, *New York Times* best-selling author, *Men Are from Mars, Women Are from Venus* book series

"The Misners understand on a very personal level how important the connection is between what you eat and your health. I met Ivan right after he was diagnosed and observed the transition from the condition of his health then to his health now. What happened for him has happened for others who are willing to make these kinds of changes, as well. It really does work!"

—Mark Hyman, MD, Director, Cleveland Clinic Center for Functional Medicine, author of *Eat Fat, Get Thin*, a *New York Times* best seller

"I personally saw Ivan's transition as he and Beth implemented the Misner Plan to regain Ivan's health. It was nothing short of remarkable. I really encourage you to pick up this book, read it, and make the transformation in your own habits to give yourself the gift of a long, healthy life."

—Jack Canfield, Cofounder of *Chicken Soup for the Soul* book series

"I watched Ivan walk through this experience with nothing short of amazement. Both he and Beth have come to really understand how food affects health in a way I'm sure they never thought they would. Beth has mastered bringing the absolute best food to your table without compromising the taste. Both Beth and Ivan have had a tremendous impact on the way I now eat and the newfound health and vitality that I get to enjoy. I really do encourage you to read this book and learn from their situation."

—Lisa Nichols, CEO, Motivating the Masses, Inc., *New York Times* best-selling author, *Abundance Now*

"I am so grateful that Ivan and Beth have learned about the gift of healing within the body through Ivan's experience. Their willingness to use qigong healing techniques as an important part of the recovery process is very wonderful. I am confident that their book will bring you hope and awareness as you move through your own experience into a state of wholeness or assist someone else along the path of healing."

—Master Chunyi Lin, founder and creator of Spring Forest Qigong and author of *Born a Healer*

"When Ivan and Beth changed their relationships with food, it had a major impact on their bodies. The transformation in their health as they became more intentional about what and how they eat has been wonderful: Ivan's regained health and Beth's regained hearing are both a testimony to the power of eating in a way that nourishes the body."

—Lise E. Janelle, DC, PCC, founder of the Centre for Heart Living and author of *Conversations with the Heart*

"Watching Ivan and Beth learn everything they can about how food influences their health has been wonderful. I have been in the front row of their journey, encouraging them along the way. I truly believe that the way Ivan's body has responded to being more properly nourished is something that is available to everyone. His experience is not a one-off coincidence."

—Eric Edmeades, serial entrepreneur and founder of WildFit

Who Should Read This Book?

My wife and I (Ivan) and our coauthor, Eddie, along with Dr. Miguel Espinoza wrote this book for those of you who have a serious health diagnosis, or know someone who has one, and are wondering if it's possible to have a positive impact on your condition with nutrition and lifestyle changes. I was not a believer that food could have any impact on my health when I received a prostate cancer diagnosis in March 2012. I knew changing the way I ate could help me be in a healthier place when my cancer treatment started, but I did not expect it would put me in remission.

The beauty of healing naturally through food, nutrition, and lifestyle changes is that all kinds of health conditions benefit from this approach. We have had people with other types of cancer, type-2 diabetes, inflammatory disease, and even cognitive problems report that their conditions were also reversed after implementing the Misner Plan in their lives.

When my cancer was diagnosed, I was told I had time to learn more about my cancer-treatment options. My wife and I used that time to research how to build up my immune system; how to engage my body's natural killer cells in the healing process; and how to induce apoptosis, or cell death, within the malignant tumor. I then developed my own approach. Within nine months, my urologist called to tell me I was in remission—*before* I chose any of the cancer-treatment options I was studying.

We had heard others discussing how it could be possible to recover health without doing traditional medical interventions for conditions such as cancer, but we never knew anyone personally who had done it. As I said, I was a skeptic, but I was curious about what felt to me like nothing more than wishful thinking. And if my urologist had not reassured me that my cancer was the slow-growing type and that I had time to research all the options, I am not sure I would have sought this path. Fortunately, I had my doctor's support and encouragement to explore *all* the options, including food and nutrition.

We also want you to know how this wonderful experience has inspired us to share our story in a way that has made the members of our corporate team healthier, and therefore, more productive, and it has spilled out into the field to our franchise owners and the members of our company, BNI (Business Network Int'l.).

This is not only the story of our experiences during this time and all the amazing things we learned along the way, but also a guide to putting our plan, the Misner Plan, into effect in your own life.

What we have learned about the Misner Plan is that it has the potential to move your body into better health, no matter what condition you may be experiencing. For example, Beth retired her hearing aids, lowered her cholesterol, and regained normal thyroid function. I lost more than forty pounds following the Misner Plan in addition to going into remission. (During the three weeks our editor was working with this manuscript, he implemented the Misner Plan and lost seventeen pounds!) Others who have implemented it have normalized their blood-sugar levels, discontinued prescription medications, and recovered from auto-immune diseases. Eddie, Beth, and I are not medical doctors, and we recommend that you consult your doctor before implementing the Misner Plan to be sure it is right for you. While Dr. Espinoza is a medical doctor, he is not *your* medical doctor, so you still need to work with a doctor who knows your particular health situation and can advise you accordingly.

There is no secret contained within the Misner Plan. You are not going to hear about a silver-bullet cure for diseases. What you are going to learn is how important your own body's immune system is and how to build it up from your kitchen so that it can do what it is meant to do: keep you healthy.

Let food be your medicine and
medicine be your food.

These are not words from a twenty-first-century alternative health-care practitioner, but rather are the ancient words of Hippocrates (b. circa 460 BCE), called the father of modern medicine.

Contents

Contents

Introduction

THE MISNER PLAN IS BORN

The visible changes in BNI founder Ivan Misner's health, his weight loss, and improved fitness level have led to request after request to share his eating protocol and fitness regimen after his cancer diagnosis and subsequent state of remission without standard medical treatments (chemotherapy, surgery, and/or radiation). We received so many requests that we felt we needed to create the Misner Plan in order to share this information with many more people than he is able to e-mail on a daily basis.

We all know and love far too many people who are obese and/or suffering from many health issues that are due primarily to how and what they eat. Many people know they need to make changes, but they are not interested in doing so. Many people want to make changes, but they don't know exactly what to do. We need support and a community in which to make lasting changes. Having the input of someone who has been there before and has regained health is very powerful.

Healing Begins in the Kitchen offers both information and support for you as you seek to regain and maintain your health while increasing your outlook for a long and healthy life. We have learned many things on this journey, and we want to share what we have learned with you. We continue to learn new things and find ourselves amazed at just how much there is to learn and understand about medical nutrition.

In this book, you will find stories of our personal experiences, struggles, and successes. We also share input we have received from other well-informed and renowned health-care professionals. As you read through the content, we encourage you to underline and highlight the sections that illuminate your own path.

Your success means so much to us. We are thrilled that you have found the Misner Plan. Focusing on eating *real*, healthy, nutritious foods can save your life and make a good life a fantastic life.

Eat real food. Enjoy real health!

Part One

THE MISNER PLAN STORY

One

A Little Perspective

Beth

As Ivan's wife and life partner, I have been preparing my entire life to support him in his healing process without knowing that exactly. My journey on the road to eating real food and enjoying real health started when I was five years old. That was when my mother discovered Adele Davis, author of *Let's Eat Right to Keep Fit* and *Let's Have Healthy Children*, and Rachel Carson, author of *Silent Spring*.

When I was thirteen years old, my mother had an experience with colon cancer. She was committed to approaching her cancer with natural therapies. She explored laetrile, high colonics, and other nutritional therapies. Mom ultimately had surgery to remove the malignant tumor and has not had any further experience with cancer.

I remember reading a very thick book entitled *World without Cancer* at that young age. I came away from this book with the concept that proper nutrition has the ability to reduce inflammation in the body, which can lead to recovered health. I read that drugs, radiation, and surgery are not the only ways to control cancer's advance. These early seeds were planted in a young girl's mind and would serve to prepare me to help Ivan find healing in our own kitchen.

After leaving home at the age of eighteen to attend college in California, I experienced freedom in many ways. One of the biggest freedoms was choosing the foods I wanted to eat.

A Little Perspective

It wasn't long before I was dieting by eating chocolate diet cookies washed down with diet soda. Slowly my diet devolved from my childhood healthy, whole-food diet to the normal standard American diet (SAD) way of eating. Once I married Ivan and we started our family, most of our meals included something ready-made and prepackaged, helping me save time in the kitchen. What I didn't realize was that the time saved in the kitchen was destined to be spent in bed with bad colds, the flu, and migraine headaches and at the doctor's office to get prescriptions for antibiotics or other medications. There simply are no shortcuts.

Along the way to Ivan's health issue, we had a couple of experiences together that opened his mind to just how influential what we eat is on the condition of our health. When our son, Trey, was about seven years old, Ivan and I began to notice him having various tics and strange neurological affects. I noticed that when he ate or drank something bright red, his behavior became aggressive and hostile. Ivan was not quite convinced that Red #40 was a trigger, but when Trey was fourteen years old, we did an experiment to confirm my suspicion that he was reacting to this food additive. I personally believe Red #40 should be completely banned from our food supply. But more about that later.

While we were noticing this about Trey, I was also seeking relief from frequent migraines, as well as chronic fatigue, adrenal fatigue, and clinical depression. I realized it was time to make a major lifestyle change. I began to exercise, following Bill Phillips's Body-for-LIFE Challenge protocol. I ate more fresh vegetables and fewer processed foods. I switched from white flour to whole-wheat flour, drank more water, and eliminated most snack foods and desserts, although I did eat a bit of fast food and drank diet soda.

Over the course of a year, I slowly lost forty-two pounds, looked much better, and had more energy. We all know that eating healthfully results in a fitter and trimmer body, but do we connect our various health issues with how we eat? I still suffered from massive migraines, but when a friend suggested to me once that there may be food triggers causing them, I quickly dismissed her input. Even though during my migraine episodes, it was all I could do to get up in the morning, drive the kids to school, return home, and crawl into bed, I could not accept that is was as simple as my diet. There had to be another cause, a more nefarious and complicated one.

I went to my chiropractor regularly. I took various supplements and herbs and tried acupuncture and anything new reported to target migraines. I even went to a neurologist for a CT scan and started a regimen of preventative medication with the hope it would keep the migraines from getting started. Nothing helped. I had been taken to the emergency room with such severe migraine pain that it took three injections of Imitrex and finally a shot of Demerol to just put me to sleep through the pain.

It was a sad and very painful chapter in my life during which Ivan could only watch with an ache in his heart, not knowing what to do. During that time a friend from church referred me to Dr. Bill Kellas and his functional medicine clinic, the Center for Advanced Medicine (CAM) in Encinitas, California, where Ivan would eventually end up going after receiving his cancer diagnosis. I quickly made my first appointment.

I arrived on a rainy day, fasting and carrying my lunch with me to eat after having the blood tests for which I needed to be fasting. I was suffering from a baby migraine that promised to build in intensity. The live-blood analysis was absolutely eye-opening. I was able to see the mold, fungus, yeast, and parasites (actually swimming around in my blood), as well as the red and white blood cells. What a shock that was. And, oh, how motivational.

After the live-blood analysis, I sat in the office with the nurse and ate my lunch: plain yogurt; organic milk; and organic, no-sugar-added applesauce—all foods I thought were healthy, but which I learned later actually feed yeast and other opportunistic micro-organisms in the body. I would also learn that one of the by-products of yeast in our bodies is methane gas, which causes pain in various ways, namely migraines. Dr. Kellas spent an hour with me going over the other tests the caring and competent staff members had done prior to my time with him that day. He encouraged me to go on his 8-Day Cleanse and then come back for some more tests and other treatment at CAM.

Day one of the cleanse dawned. Oh my. This was not going to be easy to do. It seemed complicated and difficult, and the aloe product he recommended in conjunction with the protocol tasted awful. Determined to get better, I toughed it out. After about day three, I could barely even taste the aloe juice, because my taste buds were adjusting to a massive shift. By the end of the eight days, I had lost eighteen pounds of stored toxic water and solid waste. I was never once hungry while doing the cleanse, and my energy levels actually went up from the first day. The three phases of the Misner Plan are in large part based on what we learned from Dr. Kellas.

It was after this experience with cleansing that Ivan became a little more receptive that something Trey was eating may be causing the turmoil he was experiencing. He became interested in experimenting to see if artificial color, specifically the red, might be causing the reaction in Trey. We tried an experiment.

We removed our then fourteen-year-old son from his home environment for one month to a place where we could completely control his food intake. I was scrupulous about not bringing anything that contained Red #40 into our vacation home. No chips, no crackers, no candy, no breakfast cereal, no whole-grain cereal bars, no chocolate bars (yes, even some chocolate bars have Red #40), no fruited yogurt (even peach yogurt has it)—nothing. The plan was to take him to the movies each week and allow him to have first a bright-blue treat that had no Red #40, then a bright-red treat with Red #40, then a blue treat, and finally another red treat. I thought he would surely go hungry, since it seemed everything he was eating was now being withheld from him. But we were able find other foods for him to eat.

The first week after he ate the bright-blue candy, we nervously watched both his behavior and the clock. There was no reaction at all. He remained pleasant, sweet, and flexible all day long. The second week after he ate the bright-red candy, we barely had time to notice that two hours had gone by when he became agitated and upset, yelled, and slammed his door over something relatively small. Wow.

The third week after he ate the bright-blue candy, we again watched for any signs that there was an imbalance and—nothing. The fourth week, Ivan called a technical time-out and said he did not want to give him the red candy again. He was convinced. The episode from two weeks prior was still so fresh and painful that we did not want to repeat it.

Ivan agreed with me that it was time to take Trey to Dr. Daniel Amen, author of *Change Your Brain, Change Your Life*. I made an appointment for our son to have brain scans done with SPECT (single-photon emission computed tomography) imaging, Dr. Amen's specialty. Dr. Amen said he wanted to do a brain scan without Red #40 and then after he had consumed Red #40. We all suspected there would probably be some changes in his brain function while the substance was in his bloodstream.

The brain scan done by Dr. Amen revealed that when Trey ingested Red #40, all the centers of his brain lit up, and the amygdala (the impulse-control center) shut down. Dr. Amen calls this the Ring of Fire. No wonder his behavior was so affected by this substance. All it took to get Trey's buy in was to see this Ring of Fire from the scan to understand the effect of Red

#40 on his brain. He became totally convinced and began to consciously avoid foods with Red #40 on his own, reading labels and telling people who offered him things like red-velvet cake, "Me [*sic*] and Red #40 do not get along!"

What I liked about the approach by the doctors at the Amen Clinic was that the first six prescriptions were supplements and relaxation techniques (such as tai chi and meditation), and only after making those recommendations were low doses of specific medications prescribed for a specific period. Again, seeing the results of the scans was extremely motivational and allowed us to see how much chemical food additives can affect health and behavior.

I decided that after coming this far I wanted to go even further. I changed our pool system to a saline system to reduce pool chloramines and chlorine compounds, and I had a whole-house water-filtration system installed. Ivan likes to sit in a steam shower each morning, and I was convinced that it would be better for him to sit in chlorine-free steam, as well as better for all of us to shower and bathe in chlorine-free water and for me to cook and wash our clothes in chlorine-free water. Ivan thought I was surely going over the edge at this point!

One closing observation from this time of life where everything was conspiring to prepare us for where we were heading: When I was in my midforties, Ivan started to notice that I needed to have the television turned up louder in order to hear it comfortably. He would get into my car to drive and get blasted out because of how loud I had the radio. Mind you, I listened to talk radio mostly. I was not rocking out to ZZ Top or something like that. We realized that I was having greater difficulty in hearing quiet, low sounds—the little birds singing outside in the morning, the coyotes howling at night, and even people calling my name or the doorbell ringing (thank God for my little dogs that alerted me to the arrival of visitors).

I gave in and began to wear hearing aids. It was so wonderful to be able to hear well again. I remember back to the first time I wore my hearing aids; I almost started to cry because I could hear well again.

Two

Things Get Really Personal

Beth

At the end of March 2012, my husband, who had been watching me on my own journey toward health using the alternative healthcare approach, was diagnosed with prostate cancer. This was a complete shock to both of us. His PSA had not been rising quickly; in fact, it had not even doubled in the entire time his GP had been monitoring it. Doubling time within one year is a marker that is watched for when a cancer diagnosis is suspected. The urologist had detected a very small lesion on an ultrasound scan, although nothing had been detected through the manual examination.

We were completely unprepared for this diagnosis. I was actually at CAM for my own appointment when Ivan went to get the results of his biopsy. He called to share the diagnosis with me. We had been so sure that there was nothing to worry about that I had not even gone with him to the appointment.

"It's cancer." He came right out with it on the phone.

I caught my breath.

Eight of the twelve biopsy cores had been malignant, with a Gleason score of seven (three plus four). I went straight to Dr. Kellas and told him with tears in my eyes, feeling a huge pit in the bottom of my stomach, still not daring to breathe.

His reassurance was so comforting. "We'll take care of this, Beth," he told me. "Bring him in, and we'll talk about what to do to build up his immune system and help his body get things right again."

I started to breathe again.

Ivan's diagnosing doctor, Dr. Davis, had told Ivan that he had time to research the current prostate cancer treatments, including photon therapy (radiation) and focal therapies, so he knew that he could take the time to also implement the things Dr. Kellas might advise him to do to build up his immune system.

Ivan had observed the positive impact the guidance and advice Dr. Kellas shared had on me as he assisted through the years with my specific health goals. Although Ivan was actually skeptical about alternative medicine's ability to help his body heal in this particular instance, he hoped that if he gave it a shot, at least he would be in a better place when the cancer treatment began. Ivan came straight from his urologist's office to San Diego for a weekend speaking engagement (where some of our friends circled around him after everyone had left the event and prayed over him).

As he drove the two hours from the Los Angeles area to San Diego, he formulated a list of other positive outcomes in addition to the positive test for malignancy:

1. I will experience some needed weight loss.
2. Beth and I will become closer.
3. I will slow down my work habit and take more time for rest and relaxation.

On our way home after the weekend event, we stopped in Encinitas to have a two-hour appointment with Dr. Kellas.

Dr. Kellas clearly outlined what Ivan needed to eat and not eat in order to support a strong immune system and reduce inflammation. He also suggested things Ivan could do to support the body's normal mechanisms to restore health during this time. He explained things like angiogenesis—the body's increase in blood flow to the malignant lesion in his prostate gland. Dr. Kellas really helped us both understand how certain substances, foods, and supplements work in the body and what causes cancer-cell proliferation.

Dr. Kellas explained how apoptosis, or programmed cell death, could contribute to reducing the size of the tumor and what naturally occurring plant chemicals could aid in this process. He clarified why Ivan needed to avoid certain foods for now, like omega-6 fats (in egg yolks, avocados, and high in certain nuts), vinegars, mushrooms, sugars, and red meats. He gave Ivan some very basic, easy-to-follow, and easily understood advice, like "Eat meat that comes from an animal that is not bigger than you are," and "Breathe deeply to oxygenate your blood more completely." His advice was clear. His calming demeanor was inspiring. We left him reassured and much less terrified.

Ivan had the same tests and evaluations at CAM that I had experienced some eleven years earlier. And he was also strongly encouraged to do the 8-Day Cleanse. Now, Ivan is a man who used to tell people he was a second-degree vegetarian. In other words, he ate vegetarians such as cows and sheep. To consider eating what he called rabbit food for over a week was not all that exciting to him. But he was extremely motivated. His perspective was "What do I have to lose? Nothing! And everything to gain." I was delighted with his attitude.

I had already begun to work on some variations of recipes to be used during the 8-Day Cleanse with the idea of helping Dr. Kellas and his late wife, Laurie, revise *The Toxic Immune Syndrome Cookbook*. I had been inviting a group of ladies to our home each year to do the 8-Day Cleanse, and I was having fun creating yummy, exciting meals out of the approved vegetables and grains during the cleanse for the cookbook revision. I knew that to keep Ivan happy while on the cleanse, I was going to have to keep things very tasty and interesting for him. It became my goal to bring all my creativity to the task and make the cleanse both delicious and interesting for my husband. I am happy to say he reports that not only was he never hungry during the cleanse, but also that he discovered he liked certain vegetables he never thought he would willingly eat.

I sat down at that time as well with a dear family friend and holistic doctor, Dr. Mohammad Nikkhah. For two hours, he coached me on what to cook, how to cook, and what spices and herbs to use in Ivan's meals to help his body's inflammatory response to relax. He gave me a recipe for a whole-foods juice/tonic for Ivan to drink. He also made an herbal formula for Ivan to use that has been shown to have a very positive influence on building healthy cells. He instructed me on how to perform lymphatic massage on Ivan's feet and legs and why that was important. His tips have also been integrated into the Misner Plan.

Another thing Ivan did right away was talk to several men friends in his life who had gone through prostate cancer. All but one of them had pursued radical surgery and chemotherapy or radiation. The stories he heard about the side effects, specifically incontinence and impotence, gave him the motivation he needed to seriously focus on his plan for recovering his health, if it were possible, without going to those treatments first. He did not rule them out, but he became highly committed to giving the alternative plan a no-holds-barred chance to work.

Ivan had a hard time maintaining a healthy weight with all his travel and eating in restaurants and at business dinners, and he was looking forward to being able drop a few pounds by changing his overall diet. During the cleanse alone, he lost about twelve pounds.

When he made the commitment to change his diet and eliminated Diet Coke (gasp!), red meat, gluten, sugar, and dairy, I had predicted that his weight would settle around 175 pounds. I had calculated what his ideal weight should be on the basis of his height and BMI. He was incredulous about that at the time, but he has since found that is exactly where his body has settled. His total weight loss reached just over forty pounds in the first three months of implementing what we now refer to as the Misner Plan.

He actually had to reassure our company's clients, our wonderful BNI members, and directors that as he lost weight it was because of his new way of eating, not from any chemotherapy or other cancer treatment he was undergoing. During this time, we continued to travel and eat in restaurants and at business events. We learned that we could connect ahead of time with the chefs at the various hotels in the countries we were visiting and make arrangements for organic produce, whole grains, organic rice, wild rice, and all the other approved foods for this protocol to be prepared for us.

I joined him on the 8-Day Cleanse and the follow-up meal plan, and I easily slipped back down to my ideal weight, 135 pounds. I felt that it would be easier for him to maintain this healthy lifestyle if we were both doing it. After all, what did I have to lose? Nothing! I also had everything to gain. I like to say I am doing the Misner Plan out of solidarity. I imagine it has to be easier for him to eat this way when I do, too.

Ivan began to meditate to quiet music, increase his exercise levels, and have lymphatic massage. We did a liver and gallbladder flush several times and have done many things to minimize stress, including laughing a lot, changing the type of television shows we watch, and taking vacations with friends, something we had never done before.

Five months later, Dr. Kellas suggested we take a look at the work one of his colleagues in the United Kingdom was doing with a phytonutrient extract called GC100, a concentrate made from nothing but organic plant materials that are known to have an ability to induce DNA damage repair to cells. We connected with the doctor, and Ivan was accepted into his ongoing study of the impact these phytonutrients have on cancer.

As a part of this study, Ivan had a high-definition, color Doppler ultrasound scan performed on day zero of the protocol. The scan revealed a very easily detectable lesion, or mass, in the upper right quadrant of his prostate gland. It was very dark and easy to measure with a distinct border all the way around it. It looked much like the original ultrasound scan done by his urologist in March; however, there was no angiogenesis, or increased blood flow, around the lesion. Angiogenesis starts to occur when the cancer is getting ready to grow.

He began taking the GC100, drinking alkaline Evian water bottled in glass as prescribed for the research study (and no more of the popular diet soda my husband was renowned for drinking), drinking freshly made vegetable-fruit juices, sitting in the sun twice a day for vitamin D absorption, and soaking in spring-water mineral salt baths every other day. After six weeks of this protocol, which gradually increased from GC100 to GC9000 to GC18000, stronger and stronger extracts, Ivan scheduled another high-definition, color Doppler ultrasound.

It was during this six-week time frame that we also attended the Prostate Cancer Research Institute's annual conference put on by Dr. Mark Scholz, coauthor of *Invasion of the Prostate Snatchers*. We were able to confer with preeminent doctors in the field of prostate-cancer diagnosis, monitoring, and treatment. We learned about active surveillance, the stages of prostate cancer, the various radiation treatment options, including brachytherapy (the implantation of radioactive seeds into the prostate gland), proton therapy, cryotherapy, and HIFU (high-intensity focused ultrasound). Ivan was taught how to create a history charting all the standard factors measured when someone receives a prostate cancer diagnosis and what meant what. He charted his PSA levels, the PSA-free levels, his doubling time, and his ultrasound results. He created a comprehensive notebook with all this information in one place.

Healing Begins in the Kitchen

While we learned a lot at the conference, it began to make us feel a bit alarmed again. Ivan's level of risk was evaluated to be midlevel risk, not the lowest level of risk. Having eight out of twelve cores be positive was not a good thing. The traditional medical treatments for prostate therapy are very intense and carry a high potential for serious side effects, although HIFU seemed to be getting better and better at treating without too many other complications. Even some of the active surveillance measures, such as repeated biopsies, carry the risk of unpleasant side effects, some of which may be permanent. We were uneasy, to say the least.

However, Ivan was about to have a second high-definition, color Doppler ultrasound after using the GC extract for six weeks. Just before going into the office for the scan, we got a call from Dr. LaBeau, an osteopath practicing with Dr. Kellas at CAM, informing Ivan that his PSA had actually dropped by a clinically significant amount. This time the doctor performing the ultrasound, Dr. Kevin Kelly—one of the first doctors to work on high-definition ultrasound imaging of the prostate—had the previous scan on his computer to compare this current scan with. He showed us how the lesion appeared much lighter now, almost as if it were fading. He explained this was what you would expect to see if apoptosis was taking place.

As the damaged cells were slowly eliminated by Ivan's immune system, the darkness of the tumor would be expected to lighten, and the lesion would ultimately simply fade away. The lesion would not become smaller in diameter or shrink if it were being restored by Ivan's immune system, but it would rather fade until it would not be visible any longer. He told Ivan to keep doing what he was doing. Things were going in the right direction.

We were jubilant!

During the next month, we traveled to Thailand and Hong Kong. It was intimidating to go this far from home with Ivan's specific dietary requirements and needing to travel with the GC18000, as well as our homemade granola bars (Beth's Healing Body Bars) for meal replacements and all the supplements Ivan was taking, but we managed extremely well. The hotels we stayed in had Evian water bottled in glass, and the chefs were all very engaged in preparing meals that fit Ivan's dietary needs. We only eat animal protein, other than eggs, once a day, instead of three meals per day, and when we do eat animal protein, it usually comes from seafood and very occasionally hormone- and antibiotic-free chicken. Thankfully, the hotels' chefs were able to source these meats for us while we stayed with them.

Upon our return home to California from Thailand and Hong Kong, CAM did a live-blood analysis that showed a large amount of yeast in Ivan's blood, which previously had not been the case. He started a very strict anti-yeast dietary protocol, eliminating all fruit and raw honey and taking a supplement with caprylic acid.

At this time, he went to see the acupuncturist I had been going to for help with migraines. Dr. Chen had followed the advances of a specific herb grown under very strict organic conditions in China. It contains a flavone known as apigenin that has been scientifically shown to reduce the size of prostate cancer tumors, so we added this flavone to Ivan's arsenal of supplements. We also began to eat more parsley and drink chamomile tea, two of the foods known to be high in this flavone. (Celery is also high in apigenin, but Ivan cannot tolerate the taste of celery.) Dr. Nikkhah continued to do applied kinesiology and energy work with Ivan.

All the different people on our health team enhanced one another's expertise and worked together to restore his health.

Exactly one month after the second high-definition, color Doppler ultrasound scan Dr. Kelly performed in September, Ivan went back to him for a third scan. This time Dr. Kelly left the exam room several times during the exam and checked his computer, telling me as I waited outside his office that he was having trouble locating the lesion. He needed to see exactly where the lesion was located on the scan done the previous month.

He was not telling Ivan why he was leaving the exam room repeatedly, so Ivan was quite concerned during that appointment. "What the heck is going on?" he was thinking. In the meantime, I was texting family members as I sat in the waiting room, saying, "Dr. Kelly is having a hard time finding the tumor in the scan!!!"

After finding the spot, Dr. shared that he could not find any lower outline of the tumor, and the upper portion of the lesion was just a remaining shadow. He stated that he had to guess at where to place the marks to take a measurement of the diameter because the lower edges were undetectable on the scan.

He also said in his thirty-five years of doing prostate ultrasounds with cancer patients he had never seen this result. None of his patients had used diet, nutrition, and lifestyle changes to approach their healing process.

More good news ensued as we went back to CAM two weeks after the October scan and saw firsthand that the yeast was all cleaned up in Ivan's bloodstream. Everything seemed to be hitting on all cylinders.

Ivan then returned to his original diagnosing doctor, the urologist, and showed him all the data he had gathered in the past nine months. Dr. Davis's exact words were, "This case is getting interesting!" He analyzed the high-definition, color Doppler ultrasounds and confirmed Dr. Kelly's observation that the tumor seemed to be fading, saying, "I don't understand it, but keep doing what you're doing."

The UK doctor doing the research study has said that, in his twenty years of working with people to restore health from DNA cell damage, he had not seen such an impressive and quick result. He actually formulated a GC18000+ extract for Ivan to use and recommended a double dose because of our travel-related activity, which could expose Ivan to viruses he otherwise would not be exposed to. It has been shown in scientific studies that viruses can damage healthy-cell DNA and create further DNA damage to cells already damaged and actually accelerate the proliferation of those cells.

We believe it was the combination of Ivan's dogged determination to follow the wide range of dietary recommendations made by the team of practitioners helping him with restoring his health, as well as the increased potency of the GC18000+ extract that brought this great result. And, of course, all of this working together was absolutely by the grace of God.

In early December, nine months after diagnosis, Dr. Davis let Ivan know about a recently FDA-approved prostate cancer test called the PCA3 test. He performed this test for Ivan, and his marker was twenty-six. Anything from twenty-five and below is considered the normal range for men his age. Dr. Davis's words were, "It appears to be in remission. I don't need to see you for about nine more months." This was the best news yet. We later learned that had Ivan taken this diagnostic test at the time he was diagnosed with prostate cancer, his score could have been as high as forty-five.

This test has now been replaced by the multiparametric MRI as more advances in active surveillance continue to be developed in order to reduce the numbers of unnecessary biopsies performed on men with prostate cancer and the side effects that accompany them.

Another high-definition, color Doppler ultrasound done by Dr. Kelly in February 2013 showed a nearly completely faded lesion that had also shrunk by this time. Dr. Kelly pointed out that a slight bulge remained where the tumor had been, so his body appeared to still be working to absorb the mass. It took Dr. Kelly's skilled, experienced eye to even pick it up. The technician performing the ultrasound could not see anything abnormal. The doctor's exact words were, "If I did not know there had been anything here previously, I would just go right past this. I would not even recommend a biopsy." The cells in the prostate gland appeared to be normalized at this stage in the game; there were just still too many of them in that one microscopic spot.

Ivan's choice to do active surveillance to keep an eye on the situation now moved into a different rhythm. Since he went into remission, Dr. LaBeau told him that he was now watching the hour hand instead of watching the minute hand. He no longer needed to do diagnostic tests so frequently. In a way, that made Ivan a bit antsy, because so much time passed between scans, and he wondered how things were going. On the other hand, the physical symptoms that indicated there had been something wrong (frequent urination, weak flow) were really not a factor anymore.

Ivan had been hopeful and curious about whether nutrition, diet, and lifestyle changes could make a difference when stepping onto this path. He had never known anyone who had cancer, did not pursue traditional Western medical treatment, but who also experienced healing. It has been extremely inspiring to watch his body go about the business of recovering balance and health when given the nutrients and condition necessary for health. It is our hope that our story will inspire you to join us on this path for health.

It is not easy to maintain this healthy lifestyle with our travel schedules, business engagements, and the amount of entertaining we do, but we have learned that it can be done. A new normal has evolved for us. I am writing this chapter on board a long-haul flight to Bali for a December vacation, and we have our virus-blocking face masks; a small cooler containing the GC18000+ extract jars for two weeks; a little three-ounce jar of organic, unfiltered olive oil and freshly squeezed lemon juice for salad dressing; Beth's Healing Body Bars; organic green tea bags; various liquid supplements added to water; vitamin packets; and more supplements packed away in our luggage with our H2gO alkaline water filter. We have made arrangements at our destination for spring water in glass bottles, organic vegetables, whole-grain brown rice, and seafood to be prepared in the manner we request.

Although it is not easy, eating this way is simple. It is beautiful to be in touch with how to nourish the body and view the body really as a temple, not just to view food as an emotional, feel-good thing. There is so much more to eating than just getting what tastes good. Truly, your taste buds are reprogrammed when you adopt this lifestyle. When there are baskets of snacks on the plane, the little packages of crackers or cookies are simply not an option for us. They don't even look good anymore.

We have eliminated all gluten grains, including rye, barley, kamut, and spelt because of the damage they can do to the intestinal tract. Sugar is not an ingredient we want in our food, either. High-fructose corn syrup, food preservatives, artificial flavors, and colors—these ingredients render the food item ineligible for our menu. Red meat (unless grass fed and grass finished, and then only eaten rarely), pink meat (pork), hormone- and antibiotic-laden meat are also not on our menu. You will find the entire Misner Plan outlined in detail here phase by phase.

We don't mind being high maintenance because the stakes are so high. Life is so precious, and doing anything other than living well, not simply getting through and suffering with various maladies that are avoidable and reversible, is no longer an option for us. Our friend, Dr. Fabrizio Mancini, has a lot to say about this perspective in his book *The Power of Self-Healing.* If you are just considering these concepts for the first time, Dr. Fab's book is a must-read. Simply put, the body has a built-in system for repairing and restoring health. We need to know what to do to support this system and engage its vast benefits for a wide variety of conditions.

And me? Well, I can tell you that I have no idea where my hearing aids are because I have stopped needing them. And the migraines are a dim memory in the distant past. He truly had nothing to lose and absolutely everything to gain.

What about you?

Three

BETH AND IVAN

Ivan's perspective has always been that since he is the founder of BNI, a word-of-mouth organization, he knows people are going to talk about his situation. He felt that if he were open, honest, and up-front about things, he could control the message somewhat and avoid wild speculation about what was happening. While not everyone would have preferred to be so public about this kind of a diagnosis, Ivan felt that he had no choice, given his role in BNI.

We have reprinted here the series of blog posts Ivan did from his point of diagnosis to his announcement about having been told he was in remission.

Written April 2, 2012: I announced on my social media pages last Thursday that I have a new challenge on the horizon: early-stage prostate cancer. The good news is I am fully confident that everything is going to be OK (EGBOK!), because my primary doctor made the diagnosis last week very early on in the beginning stages of prostate cancer, which appears to be a slow-growing type that is immensely treatable. What's even better news is that this type of cancer has an 85–90 percent cure rate and my doctor has predicted a full recovery for me just as many of his other male patients with this same diagnosis have achieved after undergoing treatment.

In addition to the traditional medical approach, a team of doctors at CAM in San Diego County is providing care. The treatment includes a specialized regimen of nutritional support, including supplements and other alternative modalities. One of the doctors treating me is Dr. Mark LaBeau, a [then] BNI member. Talk about your network being there to help when you really need it!

I am so thankful that this was found early, and I can definitely now speak from experience about how important it *really* is to get the routine medical exams done that health practitioners recommend for your age bracket and gender. I have learned that many times, prostate cancer has no symptoms at all, and *if* symptoms appear, they are usually when the cancer has become very advanced and difficult to treat. My doctor was able to catch this early only because I made sure to go in some months back for the routine, recommended procedure to check for things like prostate cancer in men around the age of fifty.

The results of that procedure revealed an abnormality that required a subsequent biopsy. Last week I found out the biopsy showed the presence of prostate cancer. I am very lucky that this was caught in the beginning stages when the cancer is so treatable, and I most certainly realize now, more than ever, the real importance of routine medical checkups, exams, and procedures.

I am sharing the facts about my diagnosis here today because I want to be completely transparent about what is going on and to assure everyone that I wholeheartedly believe "this too shall pass" and that I will be completely vital and healthy again posttreatment. As I've spent much of my life building relationships based on trust and teaching others how to generate positive word of mouth, I want to be sure I am maintaining the trust I've built with all those in my network by communicating honestly and directly and that I'm walking the talk to keep the word of mouth surrounding this focused on accurate information with no room or need for the invention of rumors.

I've received so many wonderful messages of encouragement from people since I announced my diagnosis on social media last week, and I am very appreciative for all the kind words. As I've said before, my wife, Beth, and I are beyond grateful to have the support of such an amazing network around the world. We really appreciate the love, and we thank everyone for their prayers. Beth and I are confident that we'll be able to look back on this as a challenging time from which much good came, and the top-notch team of medical doctors we are currently consulting with has given us quite good reason to feel strong, positive, calm, and in great spirits!

Thank you so much to all those who have voiced concern and sent me kind words of encouragement. I truly know EGBOK (everything's going to be OK), and I will certainly keep everyone updated as to how my treatment progresses. Thanks again, everyone, for all the support!

Written July 13, 2012: When I first announced back in April that I have a new health challenge on the horizon in the form of prostate cancer, many people expressed interest in staying informed about my progress, and I promised to post updates here on my blog on a consistent basis. In my last update, I mentioned that my cancer is localized and has not spread. That is still true as of today.

Over the last several months, I have been on a holistic health protocol involving a very specialized diet, eliminating toxins, and avoiding foods that stress or depress my immune system. This month, I had another PSA test done that shows no change since the first of this year. This is good news! As long as the PSA remains stable or decreases, I will continue the current treatments and assess my condition while considering other options until I am advised by my doctors to take additional actions.

I want to sincerely thank everyone who is keeping me in their thoughts and prayers—your kindness is beyond appreciated by me.

Written November 2, 2012: I would like to share an update on my health situation…I have some fairly good news. Since my last update, the scans seem to be showing a positive change. When I had an ultrasound done earlier this week, my doctor stated that he was having a hard time finding the edge of the lesion. It appears to be less distinct and much harder to identify. As these changes have been happening, my PSA level has dropped a clinically significant amount. It was rising steadily for the last several years.

I have been involved in a clinical trial using a nutritional concentrate called GC18000, produced by a doctor in the UK. The extracted molecules from certain plants are thought to have a chemotherapeutic effect on cancer. In my case, it certainly seems to be making a difference. My radiologist has been doing ultrasound scanning for thirty-five years, and he has never seen anything like this before.

I remain hopeful and positive and will share more as time goes on. Thank you for your continued well wishes and support.

Written December 12, 2012: As many of you know who follow my blog regarding my health, I have been diligently working to regain my health for the past nine months. I would like to give you another update, the best one yet!

Recently my urologist requested a PCA3 Assay to determine the likelihood that I would once again have a positive biopsy. This is a new test just approved by the FDA as a prostate cancer diagnostic test. My doctor was intrigued with the fading quality of the lesion as seen the in color Doppler ultrasound scans once I started the GC18000 protocol, which has had a swift and dramatic impact on the disease.

The results of the PCA3 Assay came back last week with a low score (far lower than the urologist expected). The physician told me it seems that I am in remission! This was certainly great news to get as we started the holiday season. I personally attribute this shift to the dietary and lifestyle changes I have made under the supervision of Dr. Kellas and (former BNI member) Dr. Mark LaBeau with CAM, as well as to the work of my doctor in the UK. His understanding of cellular DNA damage and repair of that damage through plant-molecular biology has been extremely beneficial.

I would like to wish you and yours a very happy New Year and a very healthy and successful 2013 to us all!

And that was the nine-month journey we took from Ivan's prostate cancer diagnosis to his announcement about being in remission. Some say we were blessed with the miracle we prayed for. While we absolutely do not minimize God's hand in Ivan's recovery, we don't marvel only at his miraculous quick return to health, but also at the miraculous immune-system functions which, when supported well, return the body to health so quickly and effectively. That is the real miracle. And for that we give God all the glory.

This healing capacity is available to you, too, if you will nourish the body God gave you and care for it well. It's not exactly miraculous. It is exactly what the body is designed to do!

Ivan's doctors have stressed that he needs to remain in the active surveillance mode, as prostate cancer can reoccur. It may become necessary for Ivan to seek medical intervention at some point down the road, so he is diligently monitoring his numbers, having regular tests, and watching the markers that may indicate the need to take things to the next level. In the meantime, he remains committed to his new normal, while maintaining his health with the Misner Plan.

Four

MAKING CHANGES

BETH

When Ivan and I sat down together to talk about what we were going to have to do differently, we were so overwhelmed. We knew we had to take the first step at making changes, but we did not know where to begin. We just knew we had to start. It was comforting to have the knowledge that Ivan had time to decide what treatment to pursue. This gave us the edge with implementing a dietary protocol that could make all the difference. And we had access to the medical professionals who could guide us in boosting Ivan's immune system. I decided that I needed to join him in this protocol. My immune system could stand to be boosted, as well.

We have learned that people, including ourselves, are at different places on a spectrum of commitment, intention, and tolerance. Some people want to follow a protocol to the tiniest point, doing everything recommended and being almost militant with how they approach a situation. Ivan and I realized very early on that I fall into this category.

Sometimes this is not realistic in every instance, and having an inflexible philosophy can create challenges of its own, but for someone like me, it is the way I approach challenges. I give it 110 percent and do not hold back. I typically do not cheat when I commit to a particular dietary path. Even when I was taking a free day during a twelve-week fitness challenge back in my thirties, my free day was one guilty snack, not a whole day of eating whatever I wanted.

Others are more relaxed about things, adopting a middle way that is not too extreme and not too lax. If the best option isn't accessible or possible, they are fine going with a better choice. They don't feel the same pressure that I do to get it perfect.

And then there are those who struggle with making changes and want to start with what is good and maybe work up to an option that is better, finally embracing some of those very best choices.

What is important is to approach your own life with the level of commitment at which you can succeed. If you set your sights on "best" and go around frustrated, anxious, or upset, the positive impact of the best foods is going to be offset by the negative impact of stress. I saw this with Ivan when Dr. LaBeau told him no alcohol, not even wine. We both felt that the benefit from the polyphenols, resveratrol, and the emotional benefit (pleasure, endorphins, etc.) Ivan derived from sitting down with a fine wine would be greater than the detriment of having that wine. However, having more than one glass of wine every day would have been hard on his body during the healing time. His compromise was to have one six-ounce glass of red wine every other day until such time that he was in remission. Now he has been enjoying one glass of red wine each day.

I made up three proposed health-care plans for Ivan to take a look at. One was just a bare minimum plan (good), one included a bit more (better), and one included everything Ivan was being advised to do by several health-care professionals (best). Ivan looked at it all over, chose the elements from the three categories he wanted to implement, and developed his plan. He called it Ivan's Home Health-Care Plan:

- Five-day cleanse.
- Avoid most of the inflammatory response foods, including red meat, wheat, dairy (except yogurt), and sugar, and minimize wine/alcohol.
- Drink six glasses of filtered and alkaline water per day (48 ounces) working up to eight glasses (64 ounces) for a total of 100 ounces of clear fluids, including juice and green tea.
- Chiropractic adjustment once a week.
- Lymphatic massage once a week.
- Two vitamin and mineral IVs per week at home.
- Supplements recommended by Dr. Kellas and Dr. LaBeau.
- Deep breathing exercise during evening sauna.

- Cardio exercise five days per week.
- Resistance training twice a week.

Over the course of the following few months, he made some adjustments to this plan, adding some things from the best category, dropping some elements from the plan he had created, and adding some things that had not even been suggested yet.

He had to consider his food list since there are foods that can be hard on the body during a healing crisis but may have other beneficial effects that outweigh the negative aspects. One of these foods is berries. When taking a look at the need to reduce the amount of sugars in Ivan's diet, it was suggested that he eliminate fruit altogether. Fruit is high in fructose, which gives energy to cancer cells and helps them grow and multiply. But all the body's cells need sugar for energy. And berries have such high levels of antioxidants and other healing properties that he chose to eat limited amounts of them with relish during the intense phase of his protocol, during which time other fruits were eliminated.

Honey was another food we had to take a hard look at. He felt the healing properties of honey, including the antibacterial, antifungal nature of this wonderful medicinal food, provided more benefit than harm, so Ivan used about two tablespoons of Manuka 15+ honey per day. He currently uses about the same amount and has added raw maguey (pronounced mah-GAY) sap, raw coconut nectar, raw agave nectar, and coconut and date sugars (dehydrated and powdered from the plants themselves). He refuses all other forms of table sugar, brown sugar, powdered sugar, syrups, raw sugar, evaporated cane syrup, natural sugar, palm sugar, beet sugar, xylitol, powdered stevia, stevia extract, and any other forms of sweeteners.

If you follow the Misner Plan, there may be times when your tolerance for the strictness we advocate may be low. In those times, we encourage you to use the good, better, best philosophy to make your own choices. If cheesecake is in front of you and something like fruit cobbler is also available, go for the fruit cobbler. Better yet, have a square of 80-percent-cacao organic dark chocolate. Best of all would be to have a bowl of mixed berries. Most importantly, don't beat yourself up for the occasional deviation. Where things will fall apart for you is if the occasional deviation once again becomes the norm.

Ivan and I have found that a lot of the struggle we had in the past with eating in a way that gave maximum nourishment to our bodies was all centered on habits. Creating new habits is not easy. Ivan used to watch me consult with my nutrition clients, and he told me that certain people were not likely to succeed in making the changes needed for a shift into health. "She isn't sick enough yet," he would tell me. When Ivan was diagnosed with cancer, he found the motivation that had been missing before in his own situation to make better choices and eat in the best possible way to develop a strong immune system.

Ivan and I have talked about why today's medical practitioners go straight to drugs and surgery for conditions that medical science admits diet and nutrition can correct, such as type 2 diabetes and high cholesterol. We concluded that doctors may well have gone first to those recommendations, but through the years have experienced their patients' lack of interest, ability, desire, or determination to change their habits. Doctors realize most people are just more likely to keep doing what they've always done and wish to simply take a pill!

After the AMA and American Heart Association changed the statin calculator in order to better determine which patients should be put on statin drugs, I had the opportunity to interview a cardiologist whom I asked about prescribing statins. "Basically, Beth," he said, "we are simply medicating sloth when we prescribe statins. We know that our patients are not going to be serious about making the changes they need to make to save their lives, so we offer them the drugs."

Evaluate where you are in your own life. Are you ready to begin making good choices? Are you ready to improve on that and go for the better choices? Or maybe you have the motivation and resolve to make the very best possible choices you can. With the Misner Plan, we will share with you what the good, better, and best alternatives are so that you can find your own balance in this protocol.

Ivan and I became convinced that eating a whole-food, plant-based diet was simply a matter of resetting certain habits we had developed over the years. Staying on the Misner Plan has been fairly simple, even if it is not particularly easy. We were able to create new patterns for ourselves, making adjustments where we could.

Here is an example of what I mean: Ivan loves to grill. As soon as the weather warms up enough, he fires up the grill to start cooking. Before his diagnosis, he grilled filet mignon or chicken quite often. He loved his New Braunfels smoker at home so much that he got a second one just like it for our lake house. His fuel of choice was always a particular brand of lighter-fluid-infused charcoal. It is fast lighting and stays lit once it's going. There was always a large bag of this charcoal opened somewhere near the grill and a couple of spare bags in the outdoor cabinet.

Sometime before Ivan's diagnosis, I had started quietly mentioning that I felt that the meats cooked over this particular charcoal could be carcinogenic, because they were getting infused with lighter-fluid-infused smoke. What I didn't realize was that even just the smoke from the charcoal is carcinogenic. And any of the meat that gets charred is also carcinogenic. This was something we learned together as we began to look for the substances in our diet that have been shown in scientific studies be carcinogenic.

Heterocyclic amines (HCAs) form when red meat, chicken, and fish are grilled over a high heat. HCAs have been shown to damage our genes, which raises our risk of developing cancer. Ivan realized he needed to make a change in how he grilled.

We looked into various types of grills, including electric grills and gas grills. We found a good infrared gas grill made by Char-Broil that allows us to control the level of the heat and eliminates the smoke from cooking over charcoal. We began cooking fish and vegetables on the new grill and the occasional skinless, boneless free-range chicken over a lowered heat to avoid the formation of HCAs. Ivan also cleans the grill thoroughly before cooking on it each time to avoid having any remaining meat stuck to the cooking surface become burned and stick to our next evening's dinner.

We prepare whatever we are going to grill by seasoning it and lightly brushing it with either grapeseed oil or tea seed oil. Sometimes when Ivan is grilling fish or shrimp, I will brush it with coconut oil. That gives it a really nice flavor.

As for grilling vegetables, as the vegetables blacken, the sugars in vegetables begin to burn. Any burned food should not be eaten. This really opened my eyes. I always liked to eat the darkest-cooked pancakes, toasted my bread (even gluten-free bread) to a very blackened color, and oven-roasted zucchini within an inch of its life. Ivan's experience with cancer led me to change my habits as well.

We still enjoy grilling. We just go about it in a different way.

Another place we had to take a look at our habits was at networking events: It is easy to show up to a BNI networking mixer and nibble on hot wings with bleu cheese dressing, veggie sticks dipped in ranch, minisliders, and the like. You know what I mean. But it is just as simple to have a protein shake before we attend a mixer, or to bring Misner Plan Cheesy Quinoa Muffins with us and eat a couple of them instead of the normal mixer fare. No one really cares if we eat something we brought or whether we eat at all. What's important is being with the BNI members and networking. We never knew Ivan's mantra "It's not net-sit or net-eat; it's net-*work*" would have taken on a new meaning for us twenty-eight years later.

In looking back, the first thing to change had to be our snacks. We had gotten used to eating frozen chicken strips tossed in hot pepper sauce, baked up, and served with some type of creamy dressing. I also used to make a refried bean dip from canned, vegetarian refried beans, fat-free sour cream, and low-fat shredded cheese. Canned food is not on the Misner Plan at all, because of the BPA coating on the insides of the cans, and dairy is out unless it is goat cheese with no mold inhibitors. The chips we were eating the dip with were made from genetically modified organism (GMO) corn and had, not only preservatives, but also canola oil, another ingredient we eliminated because of it being produced from a genetically modified (GM) grain (rapeseed).

I had to get creative, and I found that it was simple to switch from bean dip to guacamole. I created a quick guacamole recipe for when I just wanted to whip up a quick snack. It is tasty and very fast to prepare from all-fresh ingredients. We found a baked chip, Beanitos brand, made from black beans and brown rice and two other ingredients—sea salt and safflower oil. When I have a little more time, I make homemade crackers to have with the guacamole (four ingredients: gluten-free flour, grapeseed oil, sea salt, and water).

I make a mean yogurt dip with Italian herbs, onion powder, garlic powder, sea salt, and cayenne pepper to use with veggie sticks. I also make our Misner Plan Cheesy Quinoa Muffins and have them on hand for when we want a light snack. Two muffins can even make a handy meal for flights where we choose not to eat the airline food. Now that we have released the notion that nuts are too fattening, and we should not snack on them, we eat a small serving of cashews, macadamias, or walnuts with raisins for a snack. Delicious.

And that is another thing. As we have shifted our ingredients, we miss the Misner Plan foods when we cannot have them. I can't even imagine having scrambled eggs anymore without sautéed onions, garlic, tomatoes, and spinach or some other combination of veggies. And the gallbladder- and liver-cleansing combo of olive oil and fresh-squeezed lemon juice is our new dressing of choice. It goes on omelets, wild rice, fish, salads, and even over the Cheesy Quinoa Muffins. We like this dressing so much that it is in my carry-on bag or in my purse when we travel so we can have it on the meals we eat in restaurants.

Again, it's simple to make these substitutions, but it's not easy. You must overcome the lethargy that keeps you from doing what you need to do to switch. Once you overcome that, you are good to go.

Another thing we needed to change was our activity level. Our immune system is so much stronger when we do a moderate amount of exercise, both cardio and weight bearing. Ivan became a black belt in karate at the age of thirty-four after having been a judo student of Raul Ruiz's in the 1980s. After the intense phase of his martial-arts training, he took a break from physical fitness and only just resumed a cardio practice about eight years ago. He takes a brisk walk every weekday for a minimum of twenty minutes, including when he travels. I join him from time to time, and at other times, I use a recumbent bike or rowing machine. We both enjoy active pursuits, such as kayaking. But most of our cardiovascular exercise is brisk walking.

After receiving the cancer diagnosis, Ivan began to add some resistance training into his routine because of its value in keeping the immune system strong.

He is not a personal fan of massage, but I do Master Chunyi Lin's Qi-ssage for him in the evening from time to time, and I do some lymphatic work for him. Something recommended to us for increased lymphatic circulation is rebounding. We have a portable, folding rebounder we can travel with. Simple health bouncing for three minutes per day is all that is needed to assist the lymphatic system with circulating the lymphatic fluids throughout the body. Lymphatic circulation is improved with weight training, massage, and rebounding.

As Ivan and I took our first tentative steps onto the path of healing through whole foods, I researched online, read many books, and talked to a variety of practitioners about a wide range of topics. I soon realized that there were many conclusions out there, and a lot of them contradict one another. Have you noticed this, as well?

At one point I was sitting at the kitchen table absolutely overwhelmed by it all, and I began to cry. "What if I do something that makes the situation worse for you?"

Ivan was very reassuring and realistic, bringing me out of an emotional place to a more logical perspective. "Just get the information, let's talk it over, and we'll do the best we can do," he wisely responded. Stressing over the conflicting information and worrying over what side of it we should come down on would have its own deleterious effect on our health.

This scene at our kitchen table made me remember a section of Dr. Andy Newberg's book *Why We Believe What We Believe* where he wrote about bias. After reading his explanation of how and why we make the decisions we do, I began to see confirmation bias alive and well in both myself and others.

Dr. Newberg lists twenty-seven ways our brains distort reality through bias. I want to share some of his points, since they are important to the Misner Plan protocol and how you either will or will not find our points relevant to decisions you may need to make in your own situation:

Authoritarian bias: Believing people of power and status over others.

Confirmation bias: Emphasizing information that supports our beliefs while unconsciously ignoring or rejecting information that contradicts them.

Self-serving bias: Maintaining beliefs that benefit only our own interests and goals.

Bandwagon bias: Going along with beliefs of whatever group we are involved in.

Perseverance bias: Continuing to insist that a specific belief is true even when confronted with contradictory evidence.

Persuasion bias: Believing the more dramatic and emotional presenter more easily.

Publication bias: Accepting that anything published must be true, including publications that show positive outcomes and tend to exclude work and research that have a negative outcome.

The other day I was looking something up online at Google. I looked first for the links that seemed to support the way I was leaning on the topic. I read through them first and then read through some of the opposing views just to see if they could sway me to their side. Then I laughed at myself. I was vividly demonstrating confirmation bias!

There are many examples of how bias influences everyone's decisions relating to health, nutrition, and eating. Usually we have certain beliefs already that we filter incoming information through. For example, I know people who believe that vitamins are a waste of money. There is nothing I or anyone else can say or studies they could read that will convince them otherwise.

When we were considering whom to place our confidence in relating to advice being given about what we should or should not do, we began to understand another aspect of confirmation bias: the need to surrender our personal authority to professionals who understand a situation and its dynamics far better than we do *if* we trust those professionals.

Even when we have surrendered our personal authority relating to our health decisions, Ivan and I still retain a perspective that when the advice given to us conflicts strongly with our confirmation bias, we check in on that point and make a decision to either follow the advice or not follow it. Dr. Nikkhah was very wise in saying to me, "Ivan is the captain of his experience." There have been times when Ivan and I do not have a shared bias, but during times like that, we have been able to allow each other to have our individual biases and not allow that to become a point of contention between us.

Not everyone is going to agree with every point of the Misner Plan, and that is OK. We are simply here to share what worked for us and why we came to the conclusions we did in the hopes that you will find support here for the positive changes you want to make.

Five

IN THE KITCHEN

IVAN

When you begin the shift from the standard American diet to a more healthful, sustainable way of living and thriving, you will find that a wholesale cabinet, pantry, fridge, and freezer cleaning is in order. So Beth started the cleaning process.

I don't mind spending money, but I don't like wasting money. It wasn't until my mind-set completely shifted that I didn't feel that I was wasting money to get rid of unopened bags or to throw away half-eaten packages of food. Our dilemma was what to do with the food we no longer wanted to put into our bodies. After we had learned how detrimental to our health certain ingredients were, it was no longer an option to pass the foods containing those ingredients off to friends and/or family. The first thing we went after in the pantry was canned goods.

Rather than throwing these items away, we bagged them up and donated them to a local food pantry. We donated canned tuna, tomato sauce, pineapple, garbanzo beans, vegetarian refried beans, corn, and other canned vegetables. It still felt somehow wrong to do this, but we realized for most of the people eating from a food pantry that organic, chemical-free food was not on their shopping list to begin with.

The next thing we cleaned out was whole-wheat pasta. Again, we donated the unopened packages to the food pantry and threw away the half-used packages. After the pasta, we got rid of the artificial sweetener packets, the powdered creamer packets, the white sugar, white flour, white rice, brown sugar, corn syrup, pancake syrup, table salt, corn bread mix, pancake mix, cookie mix, brownie mix, chips, sodas, lemonade, canola oil, toasted sesame oil, candy, peanut butter, hazelnut-chocolate spread, and grape jelly.

After the pantry, we moved to the fridge. We poured out all the olives packed in vinegar, the capers, mayonnaise, mustard, ketchup, barbecue sauce, and salad dressing. We threw out the cheddar cheese, turkey lunch meat, cream cheese, strawberry yogurt, whole-wheat bread, English muffins, raisin bread, and processed parmesan cheese.

Then came the freezer. Out went the ice cream, sorbet, frozen snack foods, frozen meals, popsicles, frozen chicken tenders, and the frozen cookie dough.

Some of what we tossed may make sense to you, while other things probably are making you wonder. When we sat down with Dr. Kellas immediately after my diagnosis, he explained why it was important to eliminate all the food that would burden my body's detoxification processes and increase inflammation, such as sugar, alcohol, vinegar, fungus, artificial flavors and colors, and the chemicals (preservatives, flavors, colors, and BPA). It was very important to give my body's detoxing processes a break. When the body is overwhelmed with toxins, the natural immune-system functions become compromised. The masterful work of the white blood cells, the natural killer cells, and the T cells cannot do a thorough job. At the time of my diagnosis, I needed them all to be functioning at 110 percent.

With this understanding, it became very easy to eliminate all the substances that might compromise my immune system, including the vinegar that gives my favorite hot-pepper sauce, that deliciously tangy flavor. I knew that I would not always have to avoid these substances, but as long as I had evidence of active cancer growth in my body, I was extremely motivated to do all I could do to support the natural systems that are able to repair damage within the body and restore health. Looking back, it seems like it was a very small price to pay to have restored health and to be in remission.

Following the Misner Plan made our grocery shopping a much simpler task. Instead of looking on shelves at the many different types and brands of crackers, breads, soups, mixes, frozen meals, and the like, and reading the labels to see what ingredients we had to avoid, we began to buy the simple ingredients out of which to make these foods. Our pantry is stocked with organic dried beans and lentils, organic California brown rice, organic quinoa, wild rice, organic nuts of several varieties, organic dried dates and raisins, organic extra-virgin olive oil, organic cold-pressed grapeseed oil, organic tea seed oil, organic sesame oil, organic almond oil, organic hazelnut oil, organic cold-pressed coconut oil, organic coconut cream, raw coconut nectar, raw agave nectar, organic Manuka 15+ honey, and brown rice/black bean chips.

Our fridge has all the crisper drawers full of fresh, organic vegetables and fruits, and even the shelves are filled with bagged and washed vegetables waiting to be chopped and added to the rice and grains listed above for each day's meals. We also have our few dairy items in the fridge: homemade goat's milk yogurt, homemade goat's milk kefir, raw goat's milk butter, homemade raw goat's milk cheese, and eggs from our friends' chickens. We feel very blessed that we can buy raw goat's milk in Austin at our local farmers' market, but you may not be able to buy it where you live. Pasteurized goat's milk would be a far better choice for you than cow's milk. We also have containers of coconut milk, pomegranate juice, and our favorite home-made dressing (organic olive oil mixed with fresh lemon juice) in our fridge.

Our freezer is where we keep our grains, flours, and frozen fruits for smoothies or homemade sorbet. We also have some frozen fish and shrimp in the freezer, but we prefer to buy fresh fish and cook it the day we buy it. Some of the grains, seeds, and flours in the freezer are chia seeds, sprouted almond meal, sprouted brown-rice flour, organic gluten-free sprouted flour blend, and organic gluten-free rolled oats.

We often hear people say that they cannot afford to eat organic foods. I can tell you that our grocery list is so simple now that our food bill is actually lower on a weekly basis as a rule. When we make our larger shopping trips, our receipt is higher than our SAD counterparts, but overall, we are not spending more on our food budget. And whenever we want a snack, there is always something healthy and filling to have.

When you are living on processed, packaged, ready-to-eat, and fast food, you will spend more than I will on fresh vegetables, fruits, and grains in the long run. You will eat more because you will not feel full or satiated as soon as I will. It is very likely that your specialty coffee habit could fund your organic grocery bill. And you will spend more time than I will in the doctor's office waiting to be seen by the doctor, at the pharmacy waiting in line for medications, and off work because your immune system cannot fight off viruses and germs well.

Here is a sample shopping list Beth made last week:

- Raw goat's milk
- Goat's milk yogurt
- Goat cheese
- Coconut kefir
- Cashews
- Pistachios
- Ginger
- Onions
- Sweet potatoes
- Avocados
- Mango
- Pineapple
- Tomatoes
- Spinach
- Lemons
- Strawberries
- Wild rice
- Sprouted brown rice
- Sprouted quinoa
- Sprouted garbanzo beans
- Beanilicious or Beanitos brand chips
- Vanilla bean
- Green tea with pomegranate

Beyond what to cook, we have learned so much about the importance of *how* our food is cooked. In this area, Beth became the point person. I am not a cook by any stretch of the imagination and have often joked about my ability to burn water. My one claim to any kind of a recipe is Misner Mush, a dish I created while in college. I made Misner Mush by combining instant white rice with condensed cream of mushroom soup and microwaving on high for three to four minutes!

Please note: Misner Mush is *not* part of the Misner Plan.

Before I was in remission, Beth made a point to wait to chop any vegetables until the moment she was ready to cook or serve them. When vegetables or fruits are chopped, they become exposed to the air, and their nutrients begin to break down. This is one reason why fresh fruit juices are best consumed within ten minutes of their juicing. Oxidation begins breaking down the nutrients and antioxidants. I wanted all the benefit of those great antioxidants in my body, not escaping out into my refrigerator. Now that I am in remission, it is a bit of a time-saving technique for Beth to prepare each day's vegetables during the breakfast prep, cooking and storing them in the fridge for use later that same day.

When it comes to cooking, Beth took out all our nonstick pans and literally threw them away. Dr. Joseph Mercola writes about the safety of nonstick cookware. The conclusion Dr. Mercola makes will forever ring in our minds: "[Nonstick cookware] is perfectly safe to use, until you heat it." Well, that is the point of nonstick cookware—to cook in it. Beth had been aware that scratched nonstick pans were not good to use, but how many of us get rid of our nonstick pans when they get a little scratch, or rather do your pans, like ours used to, have many scratches, and yet you continue to use them anyway?

We invested in a set of All-Clad stainless-steel cookware, a few pieces of Xtrema ceramic cookware, and some copper pots. Beth has a couple of Le Creuset pieces, and she has her grandmother's cast-iron skillets. These are the types of pots and pans she cooks in. For baking, she uses stoneware and glass baking dishes. When she bakes muffins, she lines the muffin cups with unbleached cupcake papers to avoid using a lot of oil or butter in the cups. How we cook in these various pans is what is most important.

Our first lesson was about cooking in oil. Beth had ended her Southern tradition of deep-frying many years ago. Her deep fryer was donated to charity a long time back, but it had still been tempting for her to fill a large skillet with an inch of oil and cook up a batch of homemade chicken strips. She had to stop this practice. We learned that heating oil to a very high temperature causes chemical changes to the oil itself, and that makes it unhealthy to eat. We also learned that the smoke point of oils is critical when considering what oil to use in cooking and what oil to use after the foods are cooked for additional nutrition and flavor.

Beth generally cooks at a medium temperature in coconut oil. For higher-temperature cooking, she uses mild-tasting grapeseed oil, or for more flavor, tea seed oil. If she wants a bit of a butter flavor, she will use ghee (clarified butter) at a low temperature. She also cooks at low temperatures in red palm oil and in really fresh olive oil.

The freshness of the oil is very important when considering cooking with oil, especially olive oil. How it is extracted from the source is also important. Many oils sold in our grocery stores are extracted with solvents. These are not substances I want in my body. Refined oils often have been processed with various other chemicals and other substances we prefer not to add to our diet. We shop for expeller-pressed, unrefined, organic oils.

Steam "frying" is a very effective way to cook. The steam will penetrate and cook your foods without the added oils, if that is your goal. I was surprised by how quickly I lost weight while consuming sometimes up to one-quarter cup of olive oil per day on salads, in soups, and in our lemon olive oil dressing on vegetables and fish. It was not necessary to avoid oil for me to come into a healthy weight. Actually the use of healthy oils assisted my liver with detoxifying my body and processing extra body fat that previously had been difficult to burn off. Dr. Mark Hyman writes about the importance of eating healthy oils in his book *Eat Fat, Get Thin: Why the Fat We Eat Is the Key to Sustained Weight Loss and Vibrant Health*. We recommend his book.

Beth studied the benefits of eating raw foods and incorporated more raw food into the Misner Plan, but we did not go exclusively with raw foods. It is true that there are more active enzymes—the catalysts for digestion and complete nutritional absorption—in raw foods, but it is also possible to use food enzymes to assist with digestion. We personally eat food enzymes with every cooked meal we have. I have been eating food enzymes for many years. Probiotics also aid our digestive processes, and we consume probiotics in capsule form and by eating goat's milk yogurt and drinking coconut kefir. I definitely eat many more raw foods than I ever did before, and I enjoy them.

It is important to cook grains that have been germinated or sprouted and then cooked just to the point of being slightly soft. Fortunately, you can now buy some sprouted grains in health food stores. They should not be soggy or mushy (see, so much for Misner Mush). When grains become soggy or mushy, the growth of molds or fungi can happen so much faster. Think of cooking your grains to the point of being al dente, just like your pasta. Before I was in remission, Beth was careful not to cook extra rice, for example, and did not store any leftover rice in the fridge. The fridge is a place where the very resilient, opportunistic molds lurk. Giving molds a fresh-grain source of nourishment is a delight to them. Soggy and mushy grains have a high water content, which contributes to the faster proliferation of these microorganisms.

There are some basic cooking tools Beth needed to add to her kitchen inventory to prepare fresh foods from scratch. Gone were the bags of fresh-cut veggies (look at the list of ingredients on the packages—you will usually find preservatives in these foods), gone were the packaged grated cheeses (certainly these will have mold inhibitors, not to mention some that even contain aluminum), and gone were the frozen sweet-potato fries with their long list of added ingredients, including chemical preservatives and sugars. Washing, preparing, chopping, and cutting fresh vegetables and fruits at each meal can be very time consuming. But having the proper tools can offset this and help you with your food preparation.

The basic tools we added to our kitchen were as follows:

- Vitamix blender (with BPA-free pitcher)
- Breville juicer (both the Juice Fountain and the Juice Fountain Crush models)
- Cuisinart food processor with the twelve-cup and four-cup bowls for large and small jobs
- Fine hand grater
- Vegetable peeler
- Cutco knife set
- Yogurt maker

Beth found that it was important to wash her tools immediately after using them rather than loading them in the dishwasher for later cleanup. That way they were back in place and ready to be used at the next meal. Since there are just the two of us at home now—our kids are grown and out of the house—often the dishwasher is not turned on after every meal. It is not time consuming to rinse the bowls, pitchers, and utensils immediately after using and then wash them with soapy water while the foods are simmering in the pots and/or pans.

These tools make chopping, slicing, grating, pureeing, and blending the fresh food ingredients very much easier. They are an investment in your health, literally a health insurance payment.

Here is a cute poem Beth wrote about her new implements in the kitchen:

ODE TO THE CAN OPENER, COFFEE MAKER, AND TOASTER

You had the place of prominence
There for all to see
You got used to daily action
Feeling happy as could be

One day a subtle change came
And you weren't quite sure why
Your services were used less often
As more and more time went by

And then one day you noticed
That Toaster had gone missing
Can Opener had his plug pulled
And Coffee Maker was no longer hissing

When Can Opener was moved to the pantry
You knew it meant the end
Coffee Maker was not far behind him
She was going to join her friend

Now a new trio has come to town
Rice Steamer, Vitamix, and Juicer
They stand where you once were
They are the big producers

Let me tell you the reason why
You received a partial ban
It's all quite clear to me now
It's because of the Misner Plan!

Six

KEEPING IT SWEET

IVAN

There is a lot of discussion about sweeteners and what is healthy to eat and what is not. This topic is both interesting and divisive. The bottom line is that we try to eat things that are not processed. Beth began to use stevia in place of artificial sweetener when she was shifting her dietary habits years ago.

When we spoke to our doctors about using stevia, we learned a bit more about this product. Stevia is a plant whose leaves are slightly sweet. When stevia is used in its natural form, and the leaves are dried, crumbled, and added to tea, that is one thing. But when it is extracted, concentrated, has additives blended in, often chlorinated, and subsequently packaged, it becomes a processed substance. We have chosen to eliminate it in the Misner Plan.

Here are the ingredients listed on a popular package of a stevia-adapted sweetener: erythritol, stevia leaf extract, natural flavors, cellulose powder, and silica. Even the FDA does not consider this stevia-adapted sweetener to be stevia, but rather states on its website that it is "a highly purified product."

I would normally have no idea what erythritol is and suspect you would not, either. But I do know that the stevia leaf is not naturally more than just slightly sweet. I know that the extract is highly processed (roughly forty steps to extract from a leaf) to get something that is very intensely sweet. Some companies use chemicals like acetone, methanol, and isopropanol in the extraction process. I have no idea what natural flavors are added. I have no idea why I would want cellulose powder, but I'm guessing it is part of the product processing included as fillers or binding agents.

As a rule, Beth and I eat things that come from a plant and not things that are made in a plant, as Dr. Mark Hyman has often stated. The white powdered stevia and its companion liquid drops definitely are made in a plant. They must be altered from their natural state before they are packaged and sold to us. We do not eat them.

Here are the ingredients on the bottle of raw agave nectar in our pantry: organic raw blue agave nectar. Full stop—end of the list of ingredients on the bottle. We use raw agave nectar sparingly that has not been heat processed and raw honey, straight from a bee, which came straight from the plant. This is the choice I've made for myself, and that's the thought process in making this choice. I limit my intake of these sweeteners to no more than two tablespoons total per day, often going without them for many days in a row. I simply do not crave sweet flavors.

When Beth bakes or makes desserts, she often uses the natural sweetness of the fruits she is baking with to sweeten the muffins, pancakes, or cookies. Sometimes she adds honey, raw coconut nectar, or maguey sap. Using whole apples or making date paste as sweeteners, pureed in the Vitamix, are other ways she naturally sweetens baked items.

When we engaged fully with the Misner Plan, we found that our senses of taste shifted and went through a real change. Eventually we enjoyed our foods a lot less sweet. We also began to enjoy the flavors of a wider variety of vegetables than we had become accustomed to eating. We have heard the same comment from others who have embraced the Misner Plan.

Phases 1 and 2 of the first thirty days of the Misner Plan do not include any fruits or desserts other than lemons, so after the first month, an occasional baked apple with cinnamon felt like something very special. We had a strong focus during that first month with measurable outcomes, such as weight dropping off, pH levels balancing, and other issues correcting themselves, so it was not too hard to stay focused. Before we knew it, the first month was over, and our tastes and habits had changed. And since we don't eat processed sugars anymore, being tempted to order a sugary dessert at a restaurant or a sugary blended drink/coffee just isn't an issue. It simply is not something we eat.

Seven

WATER, WATER EVERYWHERE

BETH

When Ivan first learned of his health challenge, many people recommended that he begin drinking alkaline water, including Dr. Kellas and Dr. LaBeau at CAM. Even before his cancer was diagnosed, a friend of ours discussed her husband's use of alkaline water after being diagnosed.

Although we were aware of the recommendations many alternative practitioners made to drink alkaline water, we did not understand why or how it helped the body regain health. This health challenge has given us the opportunity to learn things we never knew we would need to know.

To make it very basic, it is really a matter of keeping our body tissues from becoming too acidic. Our standard American diet has tipped us generally into a very acidic condition known as acidosis. There are certain parts of the digestive system that must be highly acidic, the stomach being one such place, but there are other parts of the system that do not work as effectively when highly acidic, such as the small intestine where most of our nutrient absorption takes place. The foods we eat have an impact on this balance. And the balance is very important; if we are not digesting our foods properly, we cannot get the benefit from the nutrients the foods contain.

Cancer in particular has been shown to develop more actively in an acidic environment. Ivan knew that he wanted to be sure his body tissues would be in that zone where cancer-cell proliferation would be difficult. Alkalinization, oxygenation, and hydration seemed like wise strategies to employ.

I got online and researched various alkaline-water machines as well as water purifiers in general. We ended up keeping our saltwater pool, to which we had switched several years previously, upgraded our whole-house water-filtration system, and installed a reverse osmosis (RO) system in the cabinet underneath our kitchen sink. We chose not to purchase an alkaline-water machine.

The whole-house system we have uses several sizes of filters, carbon filters, crystal filters, and a UV light source. These components help to remove solid particles as well as bacteria and chlorine from our house water. This makes the water chlorine-free for bathing, showering, and washing clothes. Further, the RO system attached to our water pipes coming into our kitchen sink removes dissolved solids, such as prescription medications and other heavy metals/minerals that are undesirable to be ingested. With our filtration system, we are removing mercury, lead, arsenic, and other very toxic contaminants found regularly in municipal water supplies. Although there are safe levels of these toxins as established by the FDA in the United States, with the health challenge Ivan was facing, we felt there really were no safe levels of these toxins for him. The RO system adds back in minerals, keeping the water soft and replenished with these desirable minerals, making it quite alkaline.

Before we changed our water-filtration system, we increased the pH level of our tap water after running it through a Brita filter by either adding lemon juice or powdered coral minerals. Then we discovered the container with a small coral-sand and charcoal filter discussed earlier called H2gO and added it to our routine for producing alkaline water. After researching the various alkaline-water-producing devices on the market, our conclusion was that it was better to naturally increase the pH level of the water using these methods rather than to change it electrically through deionization.

This is another good spot to consider confirmation bias. I know that there are many people who sell alkaline-water-producing machines or who enthusiastically use these machines. I am not by any stretch of the imagination telling you *not* to use these machines or that these devices are bad. What we decided was based on our own confirmation bias toward a process that felt more natural to us.

Something that has changed for us as we move forward through this period is that we are both more in tune with how our bodies respond to various ideas or concepts. When I feel physical resistance to something (in this case installing and using an alkaline-water-producing device), I pay attention to that. When I weigh the change in my body with what physical response I sense when I consider drinking alkaline water made by adding lemon juice or the minerals, I consciously judge my internal reaction and include it in making my choice along with the facts and advice from respected consultants.

Your conclusion on this matter may be quite different than mine. You may feel a strong confirmation bias *for* the deionizing machines. I read many websites and talked to scientists, water experts, and doctors. I received a wide range of opinions and suggestions with some in conflict with others. This is true of other ideas and concepts. Some experts may tell you there is no problem with using a specific substance in your diet, while others will convince you that the particular substance in question is extremely dangerous. The more important point is the conclusion you come to personally.

During the summer of 2012, when Ivan was focusing so intentionally on increasing his water intake, he was leaning toward sparkling mineral water. He never was a big water drinker, and he joked that his favorite diet soda is actually 97 percent water. I knew that the recommendation of drinking half his body weight in ounces of water per day was going to be a difficult task, not to mention the already frequent need to use the facilities from the prostate issue. As his body shifted into a state of complete hydration, his kidneys were definitely working overtime.

After our research online into water alkalinity, we decided to test not only our tap water, the Brita filtered water, and the H2gO-filtered water, but also the sparkling mineral water, flat sparkling water with all the sparkle gone, and the Evian still water. We learned that the sparkling mineral water was the most acidic of all the waters, even more acidic than the tap water. Looking back on it now, I guess we should have known that would be the outcome because of the added carbonation, but we were certainly taken by surprise at the time. The water highest on the pH scale and the least acidic was the Evian bottled water after being filtered through the coral sand in the H2gO portable filter. And the pH stayed high after being in the refrigerator all night long. Ivan began drinking this alkalinized Evian water as his main source of hydration.

It seemed to us that the specific time we drank alkaline water could be important. Knowing that the digestive process in the stomach requires strong, undiluted stomach acids, it seemed logical to us not to drink alkaline water too close, during, or just after a meal. That's when Ivan drinks herbal tea or pomegranate juice. We learned that the stomach lining's cells will trigger the release of more stomach acid when the environment becomes too alkaline for productive digestion, but it didn't seem like we wanted to mess with that balance by drinking alkaline water with food. Again, some of you may have a different perspective, but that was how we approached this matter.

Travel was a different story. Glass-bottled Evian water was available in some of the destinations we traveled to but not all. We have gotten into the habit of traveling with portable Brita filter bottles and our H2gO portable filter. This way we can filter the tap water and drink that after running it through the alkalinizing filter, rather than drinking from the plastic water bottles that are so prevalent all over the world.

On a side note, since eliminating plastic water bottles from our own water supply, I have had far fewer hormonal imbalance issues. BPA is a xenoestrogen, and it has been linked to hormone imbalance issues in women in particular, including young girls. It is also shown in clinical studies to be linked to prostate cancer, other cancers, heart disease, and other metabolic disorders.

As Ivan's body adjusted to the new normal of proper hydration, gradually his kidneys also adjusted, and his need to visit the facilities was not as frequent. As the lesion faded and put less pressure on the urinary system, that need was reduced even further. This was a very good thing all the way around.

Eight

Know What Is in Your Foods

Ivan

A large part of what Beth and I did was to eliminate as many toxins from our food stream as possible. These toxins come in many forms, with many names and ways to hide. We learned very quickly what things on an ingredient list we wanted to avoid at all costs. The first thing we did was to eliminate any ingredient we could not pronounce or did not know what it was.

Sorbic acid, for example, is a mold inhibitor that prevents oxygen from being absorbed by cheese cells. When we ingest that ingredient, our own cells are affected and do not absorb oxygen. Cancer cells thrive in an anaerobic environment, so oxygenation of our body's cells is vital. Anything with sorbic acid or any other mold inhibitors, such as potassium sorbate or sodium benzoate, listed as an ingredient was out.

Since so many of the chemical additives in foods have been linked to cancer, we read ingredients very carefully to be sure we were avoiding artificial colors, flavors, sweeteners, any and all preservatives, aluminum, nitrates, nitrites, MSG (monosodium glutamate), high-fructose corn syrup, and the like. We got to the point where if something had more than five ingredients, we just didn't put it in the grocery cart. You may find this hard to envision, but I shopped with Beth and took good, close looks at the ingredients lists. It was very informative and enlightening.

Once we came home with an item we had not checked closely. It was simply "chopped garlic in water" on to the label on the front of the jar. However, when Beth looked at the ingredients after getting the item home, she found vinegar, salt, and high-fructose corn syrup listed there in addition to the chopped garlic and water!

Another thing we did right away to eliminate dangerous substances from our food was eliminate canned food. We learned that cans are sprayed inside with BPA (bisphenol A, an epoxy resin that exhibits hormone-like properties, as mentioned in chapter 7). The "A" stands for acetone—not something you want in your food stream. Look it up online and read about it—this is a substance we eliminated from our diet. As you know, we even stopped drinking water in plastic water bottles, choosing instead glass water bottles such as Evian or Voss. BPA is stable at room temperatures and is not believed to be transferred into foods or water; however, when hot foods are poured into the coated cans and sealed, there can be a transfer of the resin to the foods. Similarly, when plastic water bottles sit in the sun on the docks or in the transport carriers, such as trucks or trains, the same thing can occur.

Beth had a professor in college who said, "Eat foods that can spoil before they spoil." It makes sense that if we eat food that has a five-year shelf life, it is going to be difficult for our bodies to digest these foods and extract all the nutrients from them that we need. Most of the nutrients will be missing anyway. Eliminating preservatives was another step in cutting toxins out of our food stream. It just makes so much sense—if we want our health to be as good as it can be, we need to eat nutritious, digestible foods.

This meant cutting out virtually all packaged food. Beth took these changes on with gusto. She determined that if she did not make it, we would not eat it. Fortunately for me, she is a great cook and has the time to cook our food from scratch. She got really adept at making a hot breakfast for us while preparing lunch to go for me so that I could let go of the frozen meals or the hot sub sandwiches I would send out for at lunchtime. I began to take a snack for the midafternoon with me as well, something like macadamia nuts or one of Beth's Healing Body Bars. I began to eat more vegetables than I ever thought it was possible to eat in one day without turning green.

The result of these changes started with a positive drop in my weight. Maintaining a healthy weight has been a challenge for me through the years. During this time, however, I lost more than forty pounds in just three months.

This is a key component of the Misner Plan: eliminate unnecessary chemicals from your food.

Nine

The Importance of the Immune System

BETH

With all the travel Ivan and I do around the world, not to mention all the people we meet on a regular basis, it was important even before Ivan received his diagnosis of cancer to keep our immune systems strong. After we learned the added importance of how vital white blood cells are in the effort to keep healthy cells in the body, we became more focused on all the ways we could have a positive influence on our immune systems.

When we first started learning what we could about how our bodies handle cells with DNA damage (which is what cancer cells are), we learned that the immune system uses specialized cells located in the liver to summon white blood cells to remove the damaged cells. These specialized cells will also summon white blood cells to take care of a virus or bacteria that could possibly cause damage to a cell's DNA. It is an amazing example of cell-to-cell communication.

We were able to watch Ivan's white blood cells absorbing a mold spore in one of his live-blood analysis slides done at CAM. First of all, it was *huge* compared to the red blood cells! It moved like an amoeba with purpose directly toward a mold spore on the microscope slide. It completely engulfed the mold spore, absorbing it into itself to protect the red blood cells and the organs from the damage the mold might have done. It was really quite remarkable to observe.

That is all well and good to know, right? But what else we learned was that when the body is under the influence of prolonged stress (two years or more), the cells in the liver no longer call the white blood cells to do their efficient work. In addition, when the immune system is low, the cancer cells can give off signals that make them seem to be invisible to the white blood cells that happen to wander by and come in contact with them. It's like they have a cloaking device! It is so important to nourish our livers, and supporting this wonderful organ is one of the main focuses of the Misner Plan.

I asked our doctor recently what the difference was between being in remission and being cancer-free. After a brief pause, he said, "There really is not a time when a person is cancer-free." He went on to explain that we all have DNA-damaged cells that our bodies are handling all the time. When our bodies are not overly acidic and are well-oxygenated, our body is not a hospitable environment to these cells. The immune system wins, and we are less likely develop tumors or other cancerous conditions. Keeping our bodies inhospitable to cells with DNA damage is another focus of our plan.

What about protecting our bodies from viruses and bacteria? It has been noted that both of these invaders can not only damage DNA, but can also weaken our immune systems and reduce the effectiveness of the specialized cells that protect us from the multiplication of cancer cells. Protecting our bodies from viruses and bacteria is extremely important.

We all know that we should wash our hands with soap and water several times a day, especially after using the toilet and before eating. But how many other times during the day do we actually wash our hands or use hand sanitizer? What about after a networking meeting when we have shaken hands with many people? What about after going to the bank and receiving cash back from a banking transaction?

I will never forget the *MythBusters* episode Ivan and I watched where the team discovered that paper money had more bacteria than toilet seats did. Ooh, yuck. What about paying cash for a fast-food meal, and then sitting right down to eat that same meal without washing our hands? Double yuck. It is important in the quest to avoid viruses and bacteria that we wash our hands frequently.

It is also important to protect our bodies from the onslaught of viruses on long flights. The immune system can fight viruses for about three hours before the viruses will overcome our defenses. After the SARS outbreak in Asia, doctors advised folks there to wear face masks in order to keep viruses from overwhelming their immune systems. Ivan and I started wearing face masks on flights of more than three hours in duration, but Ivan found he was unable to breathe well or sleep wearing the mask.

Our acupuncturist introduced us to the iFresh negative-ion electronic mask. It is a small, personal air purifier you wear around your neck. The air purifier protects the face, nose, and mouth from viruses, bacteria, and other particles in the air that you do not want to breathe in. Since we began using the iFresh on long flights, we have not become sick after any flights or international travel. Prior to this time, we frequently returned from a long trip with sore throats or full-blown colds. The electronic mask has made a substantive difference for us.

Staying well hydrated on the plane also helps to protect the integrity of your mucosal linings in your nose and mouth, which are the first line of defense against viruses and bacteria. This means forgoing alcoholic drinks and coffee on long flights since alcohol and coffee are both quite dehydrating. If you drink either alcohol or coffee anyway, try to drink two glasses of water per drink to offset the dehydrating effects on your body.

To avoid frequent colds, we eat foods high in vitamin C, such as lemons (you can get your recommended daily allowance of vitamin C from one lemon), berries, red chili peppers, guava, broccoli, cauliflower, brussels sprouts, kiwis, papayas, sweet potatoes, oranges, and cantaloupe. When you eat lots of brightly-colored vegetables and fruits, your immune system is getting strong support because these vegetables and fruits are also extremely high in antioxidants. They are also high in other phytochemicals that are being shown in one scientific clinical study after another to have the ability to affect our health positively.

We found Dr. William Li's website, www.eattobeat.org, enlightening regarding the actual science behind why these foods have such a strong impact. Here are some of the plant nutrients (or phytochemicals) that we recruit in our kitchen to help keep ourselves healthy:

Apigenin—found in spices such as rosemary, oregano, thyme, basil, and coriander; chamomile; cloves; and foods such as lemon balm, artichokes, spinach, peppermint, red wine, and licorice—is one such phytochemical. Another is *tetrahydroxystilbene*, found in the Osage orange, also known as the hedge apple. The *ellagic acid* in pomegranates has been shown in scientific clinical research to inhibit cancer growth, specifically prostate cancer. Green tea has also been studied for its specific polyphenols. The most powerful polyphenol of all is *epigallocatechin gallate* (EGCG), which is found only in green tea. EGCG has been shown to reduce enlarged prostates and prostate tumors. *Selenium* (get your daily amount in just two Brazil nuts) and *lycopene* (stewed tomatoes provide the highest levels, while watermelon is another source) also help maintain and promote normal prostate function.

We have added some supplements to build up our immune systems and avoid colds, such as vegetarian capsules with oregano oil; Synergy's Pure Radiance C, which is simply powdered berries in a vegetarian capsule; and a zinc/herbal throat spray. The Misner Plan also endorses Premier Research Laboratories' product line. These products may be found online, and may be ordered through a health-care practitioner or from a compounding pharmacy.

In addition to these sources of immune-system support, we are also paying attention to whether we are oxygenating the body. Our cells, including the white blood cells, need to be oxygenated in order to function properly. Cancer cells thrive in a low-oxygen environment. They do not do well in a highly oxygenated environment. Breathing exercises have become very important to us. Cardio exercise has the dual benefit of helping the heart muscle remain strong and causing us to breathe deeply and oxygenate the body, organs, and cells.

Eliminating toxins in the body while nourishing the liver is paramount and is at the heart of the Misner Plan. We start each day with a liver and gallbladder cleansing smoothie we call the Sunshine Smoothie made of a whole, thinly peeled orange and thinly peeled lemon, a one-half-inch piece of ginger root, one tablespoon of extra-virgin olive oil, and a handful of ice cubes (double the amounts for two people), tossed into our Vitamix and processed until well blended. Our friend Joan Emery shared this recipe with us. We request this smoothie to be made by the hotel chefs when we travel, and most hotels are more than willing to provide it to us.

We use freshly squeezed lemon juice and olive oil in most of our meals as a liver-nourishing dressing, as mentioned before. We have both reduced our alcohol intake, limiting our consumption of alcohol to no more than one glass of red wine per day. The health benefits from red wine diminish with an increase in the amount of alcohol consumed, and the liver's ability to participate strongly in the immune system's carefully orchestrated processes becomes compromised. When the liver is compromised by too much alcohol, it cannot effectively process fat out of the body, either. The liver is critical to so many of the body's functions.

When we do get sick, we have stopped chugging cold and flu syrups (and all the chemicals, artificial colors, and alcohols they contain). Instead we drink ginger tea with honey and lemon, and a medicinal, strong tea made with black tea, cinnamon, honey, lemon, ginger, and cayenne pepper. This strong black tea is nature's decongestant. It opens our sinuses, gives us energy, and soothes our sore throats and/or coughs. It really does work.

Remember, the key to health and longevity is to have a strong, efficient immune system. There are many natural ways to keep your immune system strong and many supplements you can take, but nothing replaces eating those brightly-colored vegetables and fruits. They are perfectly designed to complement our immune systems' needs and keep us productive, fit, and healthy for a long, long time. To stay well, eat a rainbow of natural colors every day. It's fun, tasty, and effective.

Ten

Misner Plan Guidelines for Travel

Ivan

When Beth and I first started making a shift from our former eating pattern to the Misner Plan, we wondered how difficult it was going to be to maintain the plan while we traveled. With my BNI regional and country visits, not to mention the various conferences we also attend throughout the year, we rack up some serious frequent-flier miles. We had to think about ordering meals in restaurants and hotels, not only within the United States, but also in many different countries.

I have never liked to go out with people who are extremely picky about what they order and how their orders are to be prepared. It just seemed so awkward to me. Now I have become one of those people.

Our first experience with travel after my diagnosis was going to our BNI US National Conference just a few weeks after my diagnosis. Beth made contact with the conference hotel's chef, explained that I was on a medical dietary protocol, and then asked if he could prepare meals for us on the basis of our Misner Plan food list and the preparation techniques recommended (e.g., grilling with grapeseed or coconut oil and lightly steaming organic vegetables). We were pleasantly surprised that not only was the chef willing to do these things, but he also actually seemed excited to be able to go off-script a bit. It seemed like he relished a chance to be creative in a new way.

Beth e-mailed the food list with the preparation techniques to him, and he created a custom meal plan for our stay. It was that easy. No extra charge, no fuss, no stress. Granted, we were not holding our conference in the local Motel 6, but neither were we at the Ritz Carlton. There has only been one hotel in the time we have been following this protocol where we were charged extra. And then it was a simple one-hundred-dollar fee for a private, dedicated chef for seven days to prepare our meals with organically grown produce according to our specifications!

Since having that first experience, Beth created an advance sheet that she uses to work out details for our meals in advance whenever we travel on business. I have been amazed at how many times the executive chefs actually come out to meet us and say hi. They really seem to enjoy having the chance to be creative in the kitchen.

Here is a copy of what she e-mails to hotels to which she attaches the Misner Plan Foods List for the phase I am in at the time we travel:

Thank you for helping us prepare for a fantastic stay with you! My husband, Ivan Misner, was diagnosed with cancer some time ago. Instead of using the standard chemotherapy, surgery, or radiation approach, he has been using a homeopathic protocol that has taken him into remission. In order to stay healthy, he is following the medical diet recommended to him by his functional medicine doctors.

We appreciate you so much, and realize that we could not travel and maintain our lifestyle and business without the support of the kitchen wherever we go. It's that important! Out of solidarity with Ivan, I am joining him on this recommended eating plan, and we are requesting that the meals be prepared for two each day.

I have attached the Phase 3 food list to this e-mail to help you select ingredients for our meals, and then I have some suggested menus here:

Before eating breakfast (it can be served at the same time as breakfast), we need to have a Sunshine Smoothie:

Two peeled organic oranges
Two peeled organic lemons
1-inch ginger root
2 tablespoons organic olive oil

1 cup ice
Purée until smooth and creamy, serve, and enjoy immediately
Serves 2

Lemon vinaigrette is requested with all meals. Use freshly squeezed organic lemon juice; extra-virgin organic olive oil, and season vinaigrette with sea salt, herbs de Provençe, or some other dry herb blend, garlic powder, etc.

Breakfasts (please serve with lemon vinaigrette on the side):

- Veggie scrambled eggs—sautéed onion, garlic, zucchini, and spinach in scrambled eggs (1 whole egg and 2 whites), with sweet potato hash
- Goat cheese omelet—1 whole egg, 2 egg whites omelet with sautéed onion, garlic, and avocado with goat cheese
- Poached eggs (runny yolks) served over steamed spinach with roasted garlic chips

Lunches—with seafood or fowl (please serve with lemon vinaigrette on the side):

- Green salad with olive oil/lemon juice vinaigrette with grilled mahi-mahi (or other approved fish)
- Grilled vegetables (yellow squash, garlic, artichokes, broccoli, onions) with steamed white fish
- Steamed brown rice or wild rice as a side dish (pilaf recipe is fine)

Snacks (please serve with lemon vinaigrette on the side):

- Humus with veggie sticks
- Guacamole with veggie sticks
- Sweet potato "fries" (lightly coated with grapeseed oil and baked until crispy)

Suppers—vegetarian (please serve with lemon vinaigrette on the side):

- Black bean cakes with wild rice pilaf
- Veggie and brown rice bowl
- Veggie soup (such as blended asparagus soup or lentil bean soup) with wild rice on the side

Desserts:

Some chefs ask about serving desserts. It is not necessary every day, but it can be nice from time to time to have a fruit dessert (other than mixed berries) after supper. Below are some suggestions:

- Coconut-oil grilled apple or peach slices topped with a drizzle of raw agave and sprinkled with cinnamon
- Frozen pineapple sorbet (frozen organic pineapple slices processed until smooth with a little coconut or almond milk and raw organic agave)
- Frozen organic black cherries
- Baked apples with crumbled pecans, drizzled with raw honey, and sprinkled with cinnamon
- Apple crisp: apple cubes baked in ramekins, topped with organic, gluten-free, sugar-free granola and a dollop of honey-sweetened goat's or sheep's milk yogurt, topped with cinnamon

If you have any questions about recipes or ingredients for meals, please e-mail me.

Thank you,
Beth Misner
Coauthor of *Healing Begins in the Kitchen: Get Well and Stay There with the Misner Plan*

Going to restaurants is a bit different. It is not always possible or practical to contact the chef ahead of time, but most restaurants have their menus online now. We look up the restaurants in the area, review the menus, and make our choice of restaurant on the basis of what elements of the Misner Plan are already being offered in preset menu selections.

For example, if the restaurant offers prawns cooked in a creamy, buttery sauce and complex vegetable side dishes made with ingredients such as broccolini (also known as broccoli rabe) and asparagus, we know we can probably simply ask for grilled prawns served with steamed broccolini, asparagus, and pan-roasted garlic. We always ask for a side of olive oil with lemon wedges, or a fresh lemon juice and olive oil vinaigrette (I still cannot get used to the concept that all vinaigrettes do not contain vinegar, but it's true). We specify that we want no added sugar to the dressing; most restaurants add sugars to all their sauces and dressings.

Another good choice is salmon (when it is wild caught and not farmed) with steamed green beans and spinach. When we request the lemon vinaigrette and roasted garlic on the side, we are always completely satisfied with the meal. Salads are always good starters, and most restaurants have options for dessert such as mixed berries or some other type of fruit.

You may wonder if following the Misner Plan will mean you will never be able to eat out. It does mean that you will probably want to order a meal not necessarily on the menu, like we normally do, but most restaurants are fine with that. They are used to people who have allergies or other dietary restrictions and are quite cooperative. It is kind of a secret that many restaurants even have gluten-free and vegetarian menus that you may request at the time you are being seated. They are not offered automatically. You have to ask for them. You'll be surprised at how many times the restaurant will have them.

It is not always possible to find organically grown vegetables when you dine out, but we follow the good, better, best philosophy when it comes to eating organic vegetables at restaurants. It is definitely best to eat organic veggies, but it's better to eat plain, green veggies than fried or overly sauced vegetables. One of the reasons Beth and I moved to Austin, Texas, is because of the many restaurants there that source locally grown, organic produce and local farm-raised organic meats.

Eleven

WHAT IS IN YOUR MOUTH?

IVAN

After working on my immune system, making the dietary and lifestyle changes, starting the GC18000+ phytonutrient, working up to the optimum amount of alkaline water, and eliminating as many toxins as I could from my environment and foods, I began another journey into health: the dental journey.

I was referred by Dr. Mark LaBeau to Dr. Al Fallah, a biological dentist. Dr. Fallah explained how much havoc dental bacteria could wreak on my body. And I had many areas to address. Before he started with cleaning up the bacteria, he first tested the DNA of the various types of bacteria. There are strains of dental bacterium that have been linked to prostate cancer, heart disease, and other health conditions. He found the bacteria linked to prostate cancer had colonized in my gums.

Dr. Fallah got to work. Because he is a biological dentist, he has additional education in how to remove infection, toxic metals from crowns and root canals (such as nickel and mercury), and silver amalgam fillings in a way that is as safe as possible and does not create more exposure for patients. This is a very important consideration. We were advised that silver amalgam fillings should never be removed unless the patient was breathing pure oxygen and had a dental dam inserted to isolate the tooth and keep any metal debris from being swallowed and vapors from being inhaled.

When Dr. Fallah removed the old fillings, he showed me the areas underneath the fillings where bacteria had been able to grow. He removed at least two crowns and cleaned underneath them with oxygen and ozone to kill the bacteria that had colonized those hidden places. He replaced the fillings with nonreactive, ceramic material and replaced the crowns with overlays that were designed and produced right there in his office on his 3-D printer from lava-rock material.

There is quite a bit of research being conducted about the risk root canals pose to our health. Teeth are composed of living tissues with blood flow and nerves. When a root canal is performed, the lifeline to the tooth (the root with its main, large nerves) is removed, and the tooth remains in the gums, basically dead. This allows the tiny nerves left behind in microscopic side canals to feed anaerobic bacteria and excrete toxins, which leads to chronic infection. This in turn compromises the immune system.

Dr. Fallah did the painstaking work of cleaning up after a couple of root canals I'd had in the past and making sure there was no remaining infection in my mouth. This process took many months, and it had one unforeseen and uncomfortable side effect, namely lockjaw from an oral surgery procedure done by another doctor where my jaw was briefly dislocated. And it was quite expensive. The end result is that my teeth are all healthy now, my bite is correct, which will preserve the integrity of my jaw bones, and I have no colonies of nasty bacteria to create problems in my body—worth the investment, in my opinion.

Beth, curious about what kinds of health issues might be attributed to the metals and bacteria that could be hiding under her silver amalgam fillings, asked for an evaluation. Dr. Fallah recommended cleaning up her fillings and the bacteria he was sure he would find under them. When he removed the fillings, he found that one tooth had actually cracked from the expansion and contraction of the amalgam that had been used previously.

Beth had an instant reduction, nearly complete elimination, of the constant tinnitus that had been part of her everyday life for the past twenty years. Before she even got up out of the dental chair, her ears were both very quiet, and they remain that way to this day with a few exceptions that can be traced directly to her diet or a lack of sleep.

We are very glad that we pursued this aspect of our total health, even though it was quite costly. Dr. Kellas likes to say that your resources are renewable, but your health may not be. We prefer to pay with our wallets and not with our health, as he also says.

One aspect to having proper dental work done is that you are more effectively able to chew your food. Our digestive process begins even before we take that first bite of food, and the first place digestive enzymes begin working to break down the nutrients in our meals is right in our mouths. It is important to be able to chew each bite thoroughly, and having a correct bite helps with this.

Your mouth also has its own bio-zome, or colonies of beneficial bacteria that aid with both the digestive process and keeping tartar and plaque at a minimum. Dr. Ellie Phillips has written a fascinating book about how to keep your beneficial bacteria thriving in your mouth while you keep the bad guys out entitled *Kiss Your Dentist Goodbye*.

Twelve

QUESTIONS ABOUT MEAT AND DAIRY

BETH

When studying nutrition and the pros and cons of eating meat and dairy, you will en-counter many conflicting perspectives. I was raised on raw cow's and raw goat's milk. My mother grew up on a dairy farm. Milk and milk products were always plentiful and often available at every meal. I read *The Untold Story of Milk* by Ron Schmid (promoted by the Weston A. Price Foundation) a few times, so I felt raw milk and raw-milk products were very healthy, based on his recommendations.

I made my own fresh butter, incubated raw-milk yogurt, and bought raw-milk cheese. Ivan was very leery about my raw-milk habit and asked me to consider giving the kids pasteur-ized milk when they were young. I just could not stomach feeding them pasteurized dairy milk full of dead bacteria when I knew that the living microorganisms in clean raw milk were beneficial and aided in our digestion of the milk itself. Can you hear my confirmation bias coming out?

When I went through a time of focusing on losing quite a lot of weight in my midthirties, I followed Dr. Atkins's teaching and ate lots and lots of lean meat. I ate lean chicken, turkey, lamb, lean cuts of beef, and lots of canned tuna, shrimp, and other seafood. I studied the effects on the fat-burning mechanisms in the body when the body becomes catabolic versus anabolic (which is what happens when you follow the Atkins diet). And it worked like a charm for weight loss.

However, my bad cholesterol rose, pushing my total number over 200, while I dropped to a size 4, weighing only 127 pounds. Even skinny people can have high cholesterol. My ears began to ring even *more* loudly, and my migraine headaches became worse and worse. My BUN (blood urea nitrogen—a side effect from a high-protein diet) level rose, and my body began to show the negative effects of being catabolic too long. I had to pull back on the amount of animal protein I was consuming, but my total protein intake was still quite high, just under half my body weight in protein calories.

When Ivan was diagnosed, Dr. Kellas, Dr. LaBeau, and Dr. Nikkhah all advised him to eliminate dairy and meat and eat only fish, and then only the least toxic fish. With my experience forming the backdrop, I concurred, but I didn't fully understand all the potential health issues related to animal proteins.

When Ivan was accepted into the UK medical study, the first recommendation made to him was to eliminate dairy and all meat, including fish. When I asked via e-mail why that recommendation was made, my inbox was flooded with links to medical journal abstracts and other doctors' websites with their research on the carcinogenic and inflammatory effects of animal protein on our bodies. We both began to understand the damage eating a large amount of animal protein on a daily basis was doing to our health, even though it had contributed to my weight loss years before.

The only time Ivan was to eat any dairy at that stage of the game was to have a slice of hard cheese (or he could have a blended whole egg in orange juice, like an Orange Julius) about twenty minutes prior to sitting in the sun twice a day for ten to fifteen minutes each time. We call it "sun therapy." The animal cholesterol provides the building block in the body for synthesis of the sun's energy into the various forms of vitamin D. Low levels of vitamin D in the body have also been linked to prostate cancer. Since we had gone four months at the time this recommendation was made with no dairy and only egg whites (remember that I was following the protocol to support Ivan), that slice of cheese or the Orange Julius prior to our sun therapy was so delicious.

But I noticed something about my hearing when I brought the dairy back into my diet, even in this small quantity. I had been turning my hearing aids down to a lower volume through May and into June, and for the first time, when I went to have my hearing tested, my audiologist reported that there had not been a drop in my hearing. Prior to this, each time I was tested, I had lost a little bit more hearing capacity. To not have a continued decline in hearing was encouraging, but I did not link it to the Misner Plan yet.

Ivan and I started doing sun therapy in August, and during that month, I found that I needed to set my hearing aids at a slightly higher volume. I was eating the cheese with him before sitting in the sun. When we began our travel season in the fall of 2012 and were not doing sun therapy, I stopped eating cheese. And my hearing improved during the month of October to the point where I took out my hearing aids, and I have not put them back in since. I hear better than Ivan does at this point, and he hears well.

Something happened the following March that opened my eyes to the dairy connection for me. We visited the Ice Hotel in Kiruna, Sweden. Of course, it was quite cold, and the latte machine was very comforting. I began to drink two to three lattes each day we were there. By the second evening, I realized that I felt like I had cotton in both my ears. And the ringing in my head was extremely loud and high pitched. So loud that a sharp, piercing squeal awakened me from a deep sleep again, which used to happen to me quite often.

I asked Dr. Kellas about this experience. He shared with me that not only does dairy create mucus and inflammation in the body, but it also causes the openings between the vertebrae to tighten where the auditory nerves emerge from the spine and to the ears. This can lead to problems both with hearing and tinnitus. As I sit here writing this chapter, my ears are ringing loudly. I made my son a grilled cheese sandwich yesterday, and I made one for myself, too. My body seems to be the barometer for that particular dairy reaction.

Not everyone is as sensitive to dairy as I may be, but if you are having any of these hearing issues *or* chronic sinus congestion, postnasal drip, or any other type of congestion, try eliminating dairy and see if you notice any improvement. It may be as simple as that.

The Misner Plan includes a few types of nondairy milk in its food lists—almond, brown-rice, coconut, hazelnut, and hemp milk. But these milk alternatives are typically bought at the store and come in a box with a list of ingredients on the side. Have you ever looked at the ingredients on those boxes?

Some of the "special" ingredients include the following: tricalcium phosphate, vanilla extract, carrageenan, xanthan gum, gellan gum, gum acacia, natural flavors, and brown-rice sweetener.

to be perfectly honest, I'm not a fan of xanthan gum typically derived from GM corn being in my almond milk, nor do I want vanilla extract, natural flavors, or the other ingredients, either. But I had never considered how to go about making milk alternatives in my own kitchen.

I'm still learning how to do some of the things we have incorporated into the Misner Plan, and making alternative milks is one of them. I've made sprouted brown-rice milk and just learned two days ago that my juicer can make almond milk. I tried making it in my Vitamix, and it is a *lot* of work, but it sure tastes wonderful. There is no comparison between home-made almond milk and store-bought almond milk.

As a rank beginner, I would like to share my rice- and almond-milk-making methods.

To make rice milk, I tried two methods. The first was to cook organic, sprouted brown rice in my rice cooker. Then I took out one-quarter cup of the cooked rice and put it into the Vitamix, processing it with one and a half cups of purified water. It turned out pretty good, but it was also sort of bland. It would be good as a base milk for a smoothie or a protein shake. I could envision adding unsweetened, organic cacao, the scrapings of a vanilla bean, and some raw coconut nectar to have a lovely chocolate protein shake. Or I could go toward "strawberryland" and blend in frozen strawberries, a shake of cinnamon, and a little raw coconut nectar if needed. Yum!

The second method I tried actually worked a little bit better, but I'm not convinced it was the healthier of the two methods. It is probably healthier to blend the whole rice with the water. I got organic-brown-rice farina (made to cook rice cereal for young children—or people who love rice cereal), cooked that, and processed one-quarter cup of it with purified water. The consistency was much more like milk, but the flavor was still quite bland. I liked drinking this on the warm side with a little cinnamon. It was delicious that way.

Making homemade almond milk was fun, but it was labor intensive and messy, at least the way I did it! To start, I covered one cup of almonds with about one inch of purified water and soaked them uncovered overnight. In the morning, I drained off the soaking water, put the almonds into my Vitamix with two cups of fresh water, and processed them until I had fairly smooth milk. But wait! There's more! After blending them, I had to separate the almond meal from the almond milk. I found that easier said than done.

I lined a large strainer with two layers of cheesecloth, placed it over a bowl, and poured about a cup of the milk into the strainer. Well, a little bit of milk dripped slowly from the strainer, and I quickly realized I was going to need to help the process along.

I gathered up the cheesecloth and began gently pressing. More milk began to pour out, and I figured that a more firm technique would be even better. That was when my cheesecloth kind of ripped, and out squirted almond meal *and* almond milk. Oh darn, now I had to start all over. I finally got the technique right and ended up with about two cups of almond milk.

Here's the problem: it was so delicious and so amazing that I drank down the entire two cups and had nothing left for later after all that messy, difficult work! I've made almond milk this way a few more times and resisted the urge to just drink all that I made in one sitting, but I think that the effort of making it and the ensuing mess has deterred me from doing it more often.

After reading online that my Breville Juice Fountain Crush Slow Juicer can make lovely almond milk, I believe I will revive my almond-milk-making days (for the record, I love the idea of adding the scrapings of a vanilla bean and a bit of raw honey—but probably just drinking it plain would suit me better).

Regarding other animal protein, as well as milk, we have been learning a lot from Eric Edmeades, a Misner Plan advisory-board member and creator of WildFit, about nutritional anthropology and the human diet. Eric explains that our food stream has evolved more rapidly than our digestive processes have. Early humans had to work hard to obtain animal protein and lived primarily (especially the women and children) on plant sources of food. When our ancient ancestors did make a kill, they had to exert a great amount of energy. The hunters consumed most of the meat while out on the hunt, bringing very little of it back to the women and children. And then they did not have meat again for a long stretch of time until the next kill.

Eric spends time each summer with an indigenous tribe of bushmen in Africa and observes this same eating pattern to this day. Most people in the world have a totally different eating pattern. Ivan and I used to eat animal protein at every meal. If we didn't have an animal protein source in our meal, we didn't feel that we "got our protein." Going from having animal protein at every meal to only once per day, or even having a few vegetarian days in a row, has been a real shift for us. Even the type of animal protein we eat has changed.

We mainly eat eggs and seafood. Once every couple of weeks, we will eat hormone-free, antibiotic-free chicken or turkey, and maybe once or twice a month since Ivan's diagnosis have we eaten a small piece of lamb. Grass-fed (and grass finished—you have to ask about that stage, too, because often grass-fed beef is corn finished) beef is a semiannual treat, even though we could probably safely eat it more often. We simply chose to restrict our consumption because of its higher acidity and inflammatory nature.

We are learning to appreciate the high-protein levels of spinach, asparagus, quinoa, pumpkin seeds, germinated almonds, and broccoli. The word for malnutrition caused by protein deficiency is so rarely used that most of us would not recognize it if we saw it in print or heard it: kwashiorkor. We can get all our protein needed each day from plants. It takes a little planning to get complete proteins, and that is important, but feeling satiated on a vegetarian or vegan diet is not difficult.

We are moving more into the eating pattern Eric advocates in his WildFit program by going many days in a row eating a vegetarian diet (we still eat egg whites most mornings), eating seafood or chicken several days in a row, and then going many days without it.

After Ivan was told he was in remission, we began occasionally to eat wild meats, such as bison (making sure it is coming from grass-fed and grass-finished animals), ostrich, and other game meats. I do not believe we will ever eat feed-lot beef again. We have learned too much about the high saturated-fat levels, as well as the growth hormones and antibiotics pumped into the animals, that it doesn't seem like the wise thing for us to do anymore. Ivan reserves the intent to have pasture-raised, grass-fed, grass-finished filet mignon on very rare occasions, but certainly not anywhere near as often as we used to eat it, which was two or three times a week.

We used to focus on spending our times at home eating vegetarian meals and having seafood or chicken when we traveled, but Eric pointed out that we couldn't control the quality of the meats we ate when we traveled. He is right that is wiser to eat a more vegetarian menu when traveling and then eat the specific meats we want to have when we are home and can source wild-caught fish, hormone- and antibiotic-free chicken, or wild and pasture-raised meats, so that has become our pattern.

As for dairy, I have found that raw goat's milk and yogurt do not cause problems with my ears. And Ivan has been given the OK to eat raw goat's and sheep's milk cheese with no mold inhibitors in small quantities and both goat's and sheep's milk yogurt or goat's and sheep's milk kefir more regularly. Raw goat or sheep cheese with no mold inhibitors has become an occasional garnish to eggs, wild rice, asparagus, and other veggies. And it's just enough. We don't feel a desire for any more than that.

Thirteen

Mental and Spiritual Focus for Health

BETH

For centuries, humanity has known that health encompasses the mental, physical, and spiritual dimensions of our existence. But so many people alive today are oblivious to how integral these three aspects of life are. When Ivan received his diagnosis, he and I began to appreciate this connection more deeply.

Reading material like Dr. Bernie Siegel's *Love, Medicine and Miracles* helped us realize just how powerful our own minds are relating to our health. The experiences Dr. Siegel shares concerning how effective visualization is are absolutely astounding. We did not find Dr. Siegel's book until *after* Ivan was told he was in remission. I wish I had found it when we were starting the journey, but hey, at least we have it in our arsenal now.

Prayer has been a huge anchor for us. We were surprised and delighted to be prayed for following a business event the very next day after Ivan received his diagnosis. There have been other times when dinner guests have gathered around us and prayed for Ivan. Ivan has received so many encouraging e-mails from friends and business associates, letting him know they are praying for him, too. I know our faith has really strengthened us. We both have a sense that we do not walk this path alone. And we are extremely grateful that God has created healing foods and a body system that can repair itself so efficiently and quickly.

To help our respective bodies, we focus on keeping our emotions positive and upbeat. And we practice patience. Negativity has a measurable ability to suppress the immune system. When things have gotten frustrating for us, we concentrated on keeping our thoughts uplifting and encouraging, because we understood how critical that is for the body to function well and how much damage we could do with negative emotions. This is so important for anyone who is healing from some type of condition in the body.

Ivan made a firm decision to surround himself with positive influences, view uplifting and humorous television shows, and be very protective of his time off. I also became intentional about keeping my calendar full of margins and long, free periods. Since I knew I would be driving Ivan to CAM in Encinitas for his biweekly appointments (about two hours each way) in the beginning, I took a look at what obligations I needed to shift to the back burner to keep myself from being overextended. Then I made those shifts.

After I became a black belt in karate, I began to train for teacher certification in tai chi. Tai chi is an internal martial art, whereas karate is an external martial art. My tai chi trainer, Sifu Samuel Barnes, is also a qigong (*chee-gong*) master. After learning the teacher-training tai chi material, we began to work more in the area of qigong. Ivan is not an avid qigong guy, but he has experienced some positive benefits from the medical qigong I have done with him, and he appreciates it. The energetic focus is a bit too intangible for him, but the results keep him from dismissing it completely.

At one point, Ivan began to have a lot of pain in his feet. He did not realize that his arches were falling and blood flow to his feet was constricted. I did a medical qigong session with a focus on the points on his feet where the pain was the worst, and the pain subsided. When he had sleeping issues, I did medical qigong with him just before he went to sleep, and he did seem to sleep better. His attitude was so great. "It can't hurt, so let's try it."

I have included a discussion about qigong in this chapter regarding mental and spiritual focus for health because elements of qigong utilize a lot of visualization and mental focus. Certain aspects of qigong can be spiritual in nature. It has been a valuable modality to be familiar with in our journey together.

We knew before this exciting challenge came into our lives that there could be no disconnecting mind, body, and spirit. Now having come this far with all the things we have incorporated into the process, we are completely convinced that these three aspects of healthy living are inextricably intertwined.

The things I have learned during my study of qigong have been easy to implement and have had a profound impact where I have used them. When I first began to study qigong, I knew that I would see some raised eyebrows from some friends. I realized very quickly that this ancient Chinese philosophy about the body and health is one way of approaching the grand design of the One who created us with these dynamics.

Our bodies are full of electric circuits. The numerous nerves, electrical impulses, and highly conductive environment of our bodies are what make us operational, so to speak. We all have a measureable electromagnetic field that extends out from our bodies. Some people's fields are quite large, while some are much smaller, but we all have this field around us.

The premise of qigong, to put it in very simple terms, is that moving energy (called Qi) around and throughout the body can eliminate any blockages or stagnation of the flow of Qi, much like acupuncture does. There are various ways to move energy—some kinetic, some energetic. The blockage or stagnation of Qi can have a negative impact on the body's organs and system functions. Similarly, moving the energy through the body freely can have a positive impact.

Qigong may be practiced by someone for personal benefit, or it may be practiced by someone for another's benefit (medical qigong). My practice is primarily self-focused, but I have (as a student, not as a professional) offered medical qigong sessions to others. The results of the sessions are amazing. For example, while on a vacation with friends recently, one of them was thrown up into the air while kite surfing and hit the water so hard that he felt as if he had broken at least two ribs. He became progressively stiffer. His pain and discomfort intensified, so I offered to do a medical qigong session to see if his pain would be alleviated.

What he experienced after the session was amazing. He said that he felt instantly better. He went on to play tennis without pain, enjoy dinner and dancing, and was feeling good as we all retired for the evening. In the morning, he said that he had begun to experience some soreness. I did another session for him, and that was the end of his pain.

After reading Dr. Siegel's book, I feel that I understand one aspect of how qigong can have such a profound impact on health and wellness. Our minds are so unfathomably complex, and visualization is so powerful that the result of the healing work we do with qigong really does make sense. I love what Master Chunyi Lin, creator of the Spring Forest Qigong system, says: "It will work if you don't believe it, but it will work better if you do."

When we were learning about building the immune system, you may recall that we learned how beneficial stress reduction is for a strong immune system. Dr. Lise Janelle has done quite a lot of research and application of stress reduction to maximize health through the Centre for Health Living in Toronto, Ontario, Canada. We were fortunate to be able to have her gentle influence in our lives from day one.

Dr. Janelle has taught us that the food we eat and what we drink have an enormous impact on our health, as do our emotions. Love and gratitude are two states of being that soothe the nervous system and allow the immune system to function maximally. The natural state of the body is to be healthy, and it experiences "dis-ease" when there is a block to the expression of the healing power of the body. Removing both chemical and emotional toxins is necessary for healing.

You can hardly read any article on stress reduction without finding encouragement to practice meditation. When evaluating Ivan's need to bring his stress level down and learn better ways to manage the inevitable stress that comes from life in general, multiplied by a factor of at least five because of the size of his life, we realized that meditation would have a place in his health plan.

I already had a meditation practice before Ivan's diagnosis, and now he joins me frequently in meditation. While I prefer to sit silently in meditation, Ivan likes to listen to music when he sits. He brings his iPod to our quiet room, and we meditate together in our own ways. I generally sit every day, but Ivan sits a few times a week. Whether meditation is practiced for spiritual purposes or for simple relaxation, it has been shown in medical studies to build up the immune system.

You may have heard that meditation can have tremendous benefits to us both mentally and physically. It is a practice we seemed to be created to have to do—so much so that we all probably meditate every day without realizing it. I look at sleep as "forced meditation." Without it, we cannot live.

In our society today, life comes at us so fast and is so intense that our sympathetic nervous systems are usually always dominant unless we are sleeping. This is one reason we seem to exist in a chronic state of fight or flight. Our adrenal glands are overactive, and our body systems are taxed. In order to balance the impact of the fight-or-flight state, we need time in the rest-and-rebuild state. When we sleep, our sympathetic nervous system rests, while our parasympathetic nervous system is more active.

The parasympathetic nervous system is also dominant when we are in meditation. That is what happens when you sit in a relaxed position and breathe deeply, focusing on quieting the mind chatter from running through endless lists of things to do, conversations to have, and worries or concerns.

It is beneficial to our bodies, our organs, and our minds to take time when we are awake to let the parasympathetic nervous system come to the fore, while we rest the sympathetic nervous system. Studies have shown that when we spend time each day in meditation, our immune systems work better, and our blood cells are all more effective. Practiced in this way, meditation provides a significant physical benefit.

Dr. John Gray, author of the well-known book *Men Are from Mars, Women Are from Venus*, also writes in one of his latest books, *Staying Focused in a Hyper World: Natural Solutions for ADHD, Memory and Brain Performance*, about the measurable positive mental and physical benefits of meditation.

Practicing meditation in such a way that it also becomes a beneficial spiritual discipline has a positive influence on our health, too. I am very sensitive to the fruits of any particular spiritual discipline and have observed that when I added meditation to my daily practice, the fruits of the Holy Spirit as outlined in my faith tradition grew in me in a very profound and meaningful way. Rather than being leery or disapproving of practicing meditation (as some in my faith tradition are), I have welcomed the meaningful and rewarding enhancement of my spiritual development meditation has brought. Some substantial shifts have occurred in my perceptions of my experience of life. I feel more love, more joy, and more gratitude, and my physical health improves as those qualities grow within me.

To my delight, I have experienced a real weakening of the grip my ego has on my mind. I am less quick to become defensive, annoyed, and irritated by others. I don't automatically presume that the things others say are said with any kind of negative intention. It is such a liberating way to approach life.

I would like to share some basic tips on how to start practicing meditation:

- When meditating, allow yourself to be very still, very quiet, and very aware. In that stillness, be attentive to awareness itself.
- Allow yourself to stay in the present, peaceful moment. When your thoughts pull you back in time or push you forward to experiences you have not yet had, simply come back to the experience of the present moment.
- If it helps you to still your mind, focus on your breath. You might even think to yourself, *Inhale—exhale.*
- Allow yourself to move into a deep experience of awareness and the abiding peace all around and within.
- End your meditation by focusing on gratitude for all that is in your life and let that gratitude carry you back into the active world in progress all around you.

Practicing this meditative exercise daily is one way to consistently introduce a sense of calm and stability to your life. Some people are able to sit quietly like this for five minutes, some for forty minutes or longer. Find what works for you. Start with a short amount of time. Once you feel comfortable with a short amount of time, see if you can gradually increase your time to a minimum of fifteen to twenty minutes. That seems to be the optimal amount of time for a real physical and mental benefit.

Ivan sits for twenty minutes, and I sit for forty minutes. I find personally that when I sit in meditation, especially when I don't feel I have the time to do it, I end up having a different experience of the amount of time that actually is available to me. I no longer feel rushed; I am no longer in a fight-or-flight mind-set. This practice has been so beneficial that it is something we plan to continue for the rest of our long, healthy lives.

Fourteen

Ivan

Before I was diagnosed with prostate cancer, we had already implemented a few health-oriented things with our BNI staff. After my diagnosis and recovery, we realized there was a lot more we could do to emphasize healthy eating and living with our staff and BNI directors in the field.

The first thing we did was to invite our directors to be part of the beta test of the Misner Plan website. Twenty directors accepted our challenge. We were most impressed with how closely a small core of about twelve people worked together, supporting one another on to greater success. Calling themselves the Founder's Challenge Group, most all of them jumped straight into Phase 1—the 8-Day Detox.

The majority of the Founder's Challenge Group entered the Misner Plan along with a spouse or significant other. Half of those who did not complete the challenge were the ones who did not have a spouse or significant other participating with them. This seemed to indicate that long-term success with the Misner Plan could be tied in with doing the Misner Plan with a buddy, partner, or spouse when possible. This certainly was our experience. When I was diagnosed, there was no hesitation from Beth about following the protocol, even though she did not have a serious health condition. And we both benefited from it.

Most of the Founder's Challenge Group shared with us that they felt they could not have succeeded on the plan without the support of the other members of the group. Nearly 60 percent of the participants responded that the online group support was "very valuable; [they] could not have succeeded without it." These same participants told us that the inter-action with the group helped them stay on track toward achieving their goals.

This told us that there is greater success when there is support. It certainly was easier for me to follow the plan with both of us doing it. And with us both making these changes, Beth said she found it harder to eat off the plan, since she had the sense that she would be letting me down somehow.

The most beautiful thing about the feedback we got from the Founder's Challenge Group is that they were *all* willing to share the plan with others and refer those others to the Misner Plan. We have learned through this journey that there is no more powerful motivator than the personal testimony of someone who has personally experienced healing from cancer or some other serious condition through dietary changes and nutritional support. The same has been true of our Founder's Challenge Group.

While nearly every one of the Founder's Challenge Group members lost a significant amount of weight from eliminating chemicals from their diet and increasing the amount of vegeta-bles they ate, they were pleasantly surprised that they had been able to eliminate medica-tions they were taking, improve their sleep, and get up feeling rested and refreshed in the morning in addition to releasing the weight they wanted to shed.

We then invited our staff to take the Misner Plan Challenge. Nine BNI staff members ac-cepted the challenge. After just one month on the Misner Plan, they reported experiencing higher energy levels, discovered much looser-fitting clothes, slept better at night, and felt more positive and happy. It was quite dramatic how quickly they felt a positive shift.

Our bodies want to be healthy. We can substitute artificial, chemically altered, toxic ingre-dients for real, good food, and the body will continue to function. It does not function at its best, and eventually it becomes so toxic that we develop life-threatening illnesses, but we can get by for years and years. Once we eliminate those elements from our food stream, the body can repair and heal quite rapidly. I'm sure that there is a tipping point when a very ill person just cannot recover when he or she makes the switch, but I believe the majority of people who make as radical a shift as I did would experience vast improvement in their health, and many of them may experience complete recovery. It may take longer than it took me, but I believe it can happen.

One of our Founder's Challenge Group members, Mark Hackbarth, came into the Misner Plan after having bladder cancer surgery. He was told by his oncologist that he would never be rid of his cancer. Polyps would repeatedly regrow, and he would need to have surgery again to remove them. After following the Misner Plan for three months, his next update revealed that his numbers were all in the normal range, and he had gone into remission. There are no visible signs of new growths, and there are no signs of cancer cells in his blood tests at all to this day. He now believes that food is the most powerful healing medicine we have available to us.

This has been our experience, and it certainly has been my reality. It is my hope that any and all people who learn about my story will realize that they also have at their disposal all the natural healing tools I used. This is the message we share with those who work with us in our company.

Here are five changes I made at work to boost the health of my team:

1. Installed a hot and cold drinking water filtration system.
2. Engaged the entire office (those willing) in the Misner Plan.
3. Provided healthy alternatives at all staff luncheons and celebrations.
4. Started a walking club.
5. Did creative things to keep morale high in order to boost the immune function of our team.

Fifteen

IVAN AND BETH

The Misner Plan has three phases: Phase 1—the 8-Day Detox; Phase 2—Post Detox; and Phase 3—Happily Ever After. The beauty of the Misner Plan phases is that you will learn very quickly how and when to move between the phases as your health changes through the years.

Phase 1

Phase 1 is an 8-day detox focused on eating the foods that support and permit the detox pathways to open and allow toxins of all types to be released by the body. It is based on the cleanse taught by Dr. Bill Kellas of the Center for Advanced Medicine.

Our bodies store toxins in very safe places when the normal detox pathways are clogged: our fat cells, toxic water stores, solid waste in the gut, and even in brain tissue. It is possible to stimulate the release of these toxins in a safe and efficient way. This is what you will be doing during the 8-Day Detox. Of course, we strongly recommend that you consult with your physician before and during Phase 1, especially if you have any health conditions you are currently being treated for.

In Phase 1, focus on eating whole vegetables and whole grains. Be sure to eat. Don't let yourself get hungry, and do not try to fast. You need the plant nutrients, fiber, and antioxidants for the whole process. There is a two-step process to the 8-Day Detox: specific low-carbo-hydrate veggies, healthy oils, and herbs only the first four days, and then the same low-carbohydrate veggies, healthy oils, herbs, plus gluten-free, germinated or sprouted whole grains the last four days.

There are also some important supporting supplements that go along with Phase 1. Please do not try to detox without the supporting supplements, as they are designed to give you the nutritional support needed during cleansing, as well as to assist with escorting the toxins out of your body.

The recommended supplements to support Phase 1 may be purchased online from a variety of sources or purchased at most compounding pharmacies. You may have to request that they be stocked by the store. The brand we recommend is Premier Research Laboratories from Austin, Texas. You will be using the following supplements:

Base Package:

Premier Cleanse
Premier Digest
Premier Clay
Premier Probiotics
AloeMannan-FX

Optional Enhancements:

Medi-Clay-FX
Medi-Soak Cleanse
Medi-Body Bath

Instructions for the recommended use of these supporting elements of Phase 1 will follow.

The vegetables you will be eating during Phase 1 are the nonsweet vegetables. Phase 1 helps you reprogram your taste buds so that you will enjoy the great flavors of a wider variety of veg-etables, not only the sweet ones. There is no fruit (other than lemons) eaten during this phase in order to correct any imbalances in the beneficial flora in your digestive tract.

The opportunistic microorganisms in your digestive tract need sugars in order to flourish, and they will live on fruit sugars if you eat fruit during this part of the Misner Plan. You are going to basically starve them during the eight days and give the beneficial microorganisms a chance to recolonize. You will be getting protein from the vegetables you eat. The specific food list is available in the Phase 1 chapter of this book and on the Misner Plan website at www.MisnerPlan.com.

Beth has been promoting and leading an eight-day cleanse for over fifteen years. The average weight loss she has seen people achieve during the eight days is between eight and eighteen pounds. Some people lose more; some lose less. You will not be shedding fat only, which is not safe to shed so quickly in such a large amount; you will also be shedding stored water and solid waste. Yes, you will need to be near a restroom for the first three days or so.

You may be shedding toxic chemicals and heavy metals, so you might feel tired or achy. Your bladder will be adjusting to a higher intake of water than you may be used to consuming, since you will be focused on drinking half your body's weight in ounces of purified water during Phase 1 and into Phases 2 and 3.

Again, please seek your doctor's advice before starting Phase 1 of the Misner Plan. If you take medications, be sure to continue taking them, and consult your doctor about the detox before starting it. Your medications may need to be adjusted as your body chemistry changes during the 8-Day Detox. One of our type-2 diabetic Misner Planners reported that after day three of Phase 1, his doctor advised him to reduce the amount of insulin he was using. By day eight, he no longer needed to use any insulin at all. We emphasize this: stay in close contact with your health-care practitioner before, during, and after Phase 1.

If you are experiencing serious health issues, after consulting your doctor, you have the choice to start in the Misner Plan with Phase 1 or Phase 2. Some people should *not* attempt Phase 1. They are women who are pregnant or breastfeeding, those with type-1 diabetes (insulin dependent), those with advanced cancer who are losing weight rapidly, and those taking a medication for preventing blood clots, heart arrhythmia, or convulsions. Anyone who is struggling with adrenal exhaustion will need to be supervised by a doctor during Phase 1. If you are in this condition, please do not try to do Phase 1 on your own. Contact us through the Misner Plan website for a referral to a Misner-Plan certified health coach who can guide you through the appropriate process for your condition.

There will be times during the first year and beyond when you will want to repeat Phase 1 in its entirety or simply do a mini detox. Doing a four-day mini detox after long trips or vacations works great to fine-tune the body and maintain ultimate health.

You will be testing your pH levels throughout Phase 1. We have information here to help you understand the importance of this part of Phase 1 and how to do it properly:

Adapted from *Healthy Kitchen, Healthy Body by* Dr. Bill and Laurie Kellas, Andrea Dworkin, and Beth Misner: Testing your pH level, or relative acidity or alkalinity, is important during Phase 1. It is a simple and relatively accurate way to monitor for possible fermentation of undigested foods in the gut and the resulting overall body toxicity this can cause. It may help you learn what foods your body tolerates well and how that changes as your health changes. The pH of the urine can help provide this information. Some people test their saliva pH, but there are so many variables that can change your reading that checking the urine pH for the most accuracy is preferred.

It is very important to test your urine first thing in the morning with pH strips that have a test range between 4.5 and 7.5. Waiting too late in the day can give you an elevated pH reading. Briefly dip a one- to two-inch strip of the pH paper into the urine stream toward the end of your first urination after sunrise. If the sample is taken at the beginning of urination, there may be sediment being excreted, which can give you a false pH reading. This sediment is naturally quite acidic. If you have voided your bladder during the night after 3:00 a.m., you may dip the strip into your urine stream right away.

Compare the color of the wet part of the strip with the color guide on the pH strip dispenser to get your reading. It is a good idea to keep a record of your diet one day and your urine pH the next day to establish a connection between what you eat and how it affects your urine pH.

Optimal first-morning urine pH should be between 5.8 and 6.2. A reading that is higher than 6.2 may indicate fermentation or an allergy to food, and certain foods should be reduced or eliminated from your diet until your health, and therefore your digestion, improves. Some experimentation can narrow down exactly which foods are causing the problem. A reading that is below 5.8 can also indicate fermentation in a different stage. When fermentation is happening in the gut, the pH can rise and then suddenly drop as the body produces a vinegar-like substance. A low reading may also indicate chemical/pesticide/heavy metal toxicity or a mineral deficiency. Premier Research Laboratories' Medi-Body Bath was specifically formulated to aid the body in releasing these particular toxins through the detox pathway of your skin.

As you go through Phase 1, you will notice that your pH number will fluctuate. Some days it may be very low, and other days it may be very high. As you continue following the 8-Day Detox instructions, it should settle into the optimal range. If it does not, there may be additional detoxing you could consider doing, such as oral or IV chelation, a sauna detox program, or a liver flush.

As your health improves, you will probably be able to tolerate more foods and eat them more often with no negative impact on your body chemistry. If your urine pH stays in the normal range for five consecutive days after eating certain foods, those foods can most likely be consumed on a more regular basis. This is especially important to note as you transition from Phase 2 to Phase 3 of the Misner Plan. If your urine pH is not yet in the optimal range, we would encourage you to remain in Phase 2 longer than the first thirty days until your pH is between 5.8 and 6.2. You can repeat the Phase 1/Phase 2 cycle up to three times safely, but do not try to do Phase 1 longer than the eight days. Your body needs to rest between cleanses.

Test your urine daily for the eight-day period and then once per week to keep an accurate pH diary. As mentioned before, if you see a spike or drop in your pH, look back in your food journal to the day before to identify what might have caused it. A spike could be caused by a higher-carbohydrate food feeding opportunistic (bad) bacteria. A drop could be caused by ingesting food additives or chemicals such as preservatives, natural flavors, or pesticides from conventionally grown produce that has been improperly washed.

If, for example, you have ideal urine pH the day after eating peas or carrots, they can then be eaten in moderation. As your health approaches an optimal level, most foods will be tolerated well without causing a change in your pH, and then even a sugar-free dessert occasionally won't be a problem.

If you tend to eat a lot of a specific food, like any of our Misner Plan desserts or extra fruit, you may notice a change in your pH numbers. That may be an indication that you should slow down with those foods or completely eliminate them for a while until you are back in a healthy pH range for at least five days.

The lower the carbohydrate content, the less likely the vegetable is to ferment. Carbohydrate content of vegetables should also be taken into consideration when balancing carbohydrates, protein, and vegetables in a 20/30/20/30 ratio. You will also want to add back foods with lower sugar content as your urine pH stays consistently at 6 (plus or minus .2). If it goes up, do not move into the next carbohydrate category.

We have created lists for you to refer to as you move from Phase 2 to Phase 3:

3 Percent Carbohydrate Content Vegetables
Asparagus
Bamboo shoots
Beet greens
Bean sprouts
Broccoli
Cabbage
Cauliflower
Celery
Chard
Cucumber
Lettuce
Mushrooms
Mustard greens
Parsley
Radishes
Sauerkraut
Squash, summer
Turnip tops
Watercress

6 Percent Carbohydrate Vegetables
Beans, green
Beans, wax
Eggplant
Leeks
Parsley
Okra

Pepper, green
Pepper, red
Pumpkin
Squash, winter
Tomatoes
Turnips

6 Percent Carbohydrate Fruits
Cantaloupe
Honeydew
Watermelon
Strawberries

9 Percent Carbohydrate Vegetables
Artichokes
Beets
Brussels sprouts
Carrots
Onions
Rutabagas

9 Percent Carbohydrate Fruits
Blackberries
Cranberries
Currants
Grapefruit
Lemons
Limes
Papaya
Tangerines
Gooseberries

12 Percent Carbohydrate Vegetables
Beans, red
Kidney beans, canned
Peas

12 Percent Carbohydrate Fruits
Apples
Blueberries
Huckleberries
Mangoes
Nectarines
Pears

15 Percent Carbohydrate Vegetables
Soybeans, dry (non-GMO)

15 Percent Carbohydrate Fruits
Cherries, sour
Loganberries
Oranges
Peaches
Pineapple
Plums
Raspberries

18 Percent Carbohydrate Vegetables
Horseradish
Potatoes

18 Percent Carbohydrate Fruits
Cherries, sweet
Crabapples
Figs, fresh
Pomegranates
Grapes

21 Percent Carbohydrate Vegetables
Beans, lima, fresh
Corn, fresh (non-GMO)

21 Percent Carbohydrate Fruits
Banana
Prunes

Phase 2

Phase 2 begins with day nine and goes to day thirty immediately after Phase 1. You will be eating all the same vegetables and grains you ate while doing the 8-Day Detox, and you will add some animal protein sources. We recommend that you continue taking the Premier Research Laboratories' supplements into Phase 2 and beyond on a slightly different schedule. The ingredients of these whole-food supplements will continue to support building the immune system and removing everyday toxins.

You will be eating whole-food, mostly plant-based meals. You may wish to eat Phase 2 meats rarely, every couple of weeks, or maybe not at all. The list of Phase 2 foods is also available at the www.MisnerPlan.com and in the Phase 2 chapter of this book.

Depending on how your body responds to Phase 1, you may wish to stay in Phase 2 longer than the rest of the month. You may wish to spend two to three months in this phase. It is a very effective phase for eliminating cravings, moving into full health for those who have major issues or who use multiple medications, and for those who have a lot of weight to shed. Ivan stayed in Phase 2 for six months after he was told he was in remission from cancer, bringing the total time he spent in Phase 2 to a full two years!

Some indications that you may need to stay in Phase 2 longer include the following:

- A urine pH that is not in the ideal range after completing Phase 2 for the first time.
- A desire to continue shedding excess weight until your body reaches its ideal weight and percentage of body fat.
- You're still dealing with other health issues that have not yet resolved themselves, such as high blood pressure, high blood sugar, low energy, and migraines.

With your health-care practitioner's guidance, you can decide when you are ready to move into Phase 3.

If you are basically in pretty good health, or you cannot take several days off where you may feel a bit weak and puny, you may choose to start on the Misner Plan in Phase 2. You will move just a little more slowly into health, but there is nothing wrong with that. It will be a steady, sure progression from where you are now to where you want to be. With the addition of the appropriate supplements and the Phase 2 food list, your body will still be able to do a slow detox.

Phase 3

The food list for Phase 3 is quite a bit longer and may be found at www.MisnerPlan.com and in the Phase 3 chapter of this book. At this point you will be able to enjoy some additions like gluten-free bread; homemade, gluten-free pancakes; some fruit-based desserts; and the sweeter vegetables, such as beets, carrots, tomatoes, and jicama. And you can also add back in delicious, antioxidant-rich fruit. You will be able to use natural sweeteners like raw honey, maguey sap, raw coconut nectar, and raw agave nectar. Baking with a gluten-free-flour mix and eating nut butters will be part of your routine.

It is during Phase 3 that you can have something quite special. That may range from New Zealand lamb to a small portion of 80-percent-plus-cacao organic dark chocolate. You can wisely select certain foods that have labels and lists of ingredients. You have reset your cravings, your blood-sugar levels, and your intestinal flora. You have landed at your ideal weight and will maintain that effortlessly, even when you travel. You will have redefined what good food is, and when you stray, you will feel it immediately. You will remain motivated to stay on the Misner Plan happily ever after. It will become your new normal.

Postscript from Ivan:

I posted this announcement on my October 21, 2013, blog. It makes a fitting close to this part of our journey.

> If you had told me two years ago when I was diagnosed with prostate cancer that today I would be reveling in the news of a clean bill of health, I wouldn't have believed you. However, I recently received a report from my radiologist stating that there is "gross remission of the prostate cancer...with no gross evidence of malignancy remaining." In other words, a clean bill of health is exactly what I now

have, and I owe it largely to the radical changes I made in my diet and my eating habits.

In addition to this report from Dr. Kelly, I also had the results of my subsequent PCA3 test come back well within the normal range for a man my age with a score of 17. Just under a year ago earlier, my projected score was 45. My most recent PCA3 test result was 13.

The Misner Plan is my new normal. I hope my experience is helpful in some way for your particular journey. Please remember to find a doctor who can work with you as you focus on recapturing and maintaining your health and wellness.

Part Two

EDUCATIONAL CONTENT

Sixteen

We Are Nuts about Nuts

Ivan and Beth

Nuts are very healthy foods and are full of beneficial macronutrients and micronutrients, not to mention fiber for bowel regulation. What most people do not realize is that all nuts also contain antinutrients in the form of many different types of protective substances that work very hard to keep the plant's seed intact so that it can germinate after passing through the animal or person who ate it. Eric Edmeades teaches this in his WildFit program, and Sally Fallon writes about it extensively in *Nourishing Traditions*.

Nuts, grains, and beans are plant seeds, so they all have to be specially prepped before we eat them—not only so we can digest them and receive the benefit from their nutritious composition, but also so they do not harm us by creating dysbiosis through binding to other nutrients from other foods we eat at the same time. Dysbiosis is the condition that arises when your gut flora, the beneficial bacteria that aid in the digestive process, gets out of balance, and opportunistic bacteria begin to overgrow.

Antinutrients can actually cause digestive stress, reduce our ability to absorb minerals, and stop important enzymatic processes. It is not enough to boil them for long periods, in the case of legumes and grains, or roast them, in the case of nuts, to get them ready to eat. Only soaking them starts the germination process, which releases the antinutrients and allows your body to metabolize all the beneficial nutrients available in these tasty foods. You do not need to leave them in the soaking water so long that you see the sprout emerging. Specific instructions for the various types of seeds and beans will follow.

Phytic Acid

One antinutrient is phytic acid that can block protein absorption, not only from the seed, nut, or bean itself, but also from any other protein source eaten with the food. Eating these foods before neutralizing phytic acid, which is an enzyme inhibitor, can create mineral deficiencies.

Oligosaccharides

Hard beans, such as kidney, navy, and black beans, contain complex sugars called oligosaccharides. We do not produce the enzyme necessary to break down these sugars, and so they lead to fermentation in the gut, a condition we seek to eliminate when detoxing the body.

Saponins

Quinoa seeds are coated with saponin, a bitter-tasting chemical compound also found on soybeans, chickpeas, mung beans, and lentils. While not considered to be toxic to humans, saponins impart a quite bitter flavor that is not well tolerated by some people. A quick rinse before soaking will help to remove the saponins. You may notice that the rinse water becomes foamy—saponin is used as a detergent in some cultures because of its soapy nature. It is possible to purchase quinoa that has been rinsed, or you may also forgo rinsing if your palate is not offended by the taste from the saponins. If you buy sprouted quinoa, it is not necessary to remove any saponins, as they will already have been washed away.

Instructions for Soaking

Soaking seeds, nuts, and beans before cooking and eating them is necessary for optimal health as well as detoxification. They truly cannot be considered to be edible without soaking. In reality, they are not, because you cannot digest them. For much more on this topic, we recommend reading Sally Fallon's *Nourishing Traditions*.

For our busy lives, we have found that there are quite a few sprouted options available in stores today, such as sprouted quinoa (as mentioned), sprouted brown rice, and sprouted nuts; however, it is easy to prepare them in your own home. It just takes planning a day or two before you want to eat them.

The seeds need to be soaked in purified warm water with the water poured off a couple of times and fresh water used during the soaking process. Be sure to use glass or ceramic bowls, not metal or plastic.

LEGUMES

The antinutrients in legumes take quite some time to be released when soaking, and you will not be able to reduce them completely through germination. We recommend soaking beans for a couple of days. If you choose to soak on the stove and not in an electric pot on a very low setting to keep them at 150°F, please watch your water levels closely, especially during the first five to six hours, in order to not burn the beans. Add one teaspoon of baking soda to beans that are covered with about one inch of water and stir gently. We recommend that you replace the water a couple of times. Be sure to add one teaspoon of baking soda each time you change the water. Germinating your beans will shorten their cooking time, if you go straight from soaking to cooking.

Once done soaking, you can rinse, refresh the water, and cook until soft, about thirty to forty minutes, depending on the quantity you are preparing.

NUTS AND SEEDS

These have less phytic acid but are relatively high in enzyme inhibitors, so you will want to add one teaspoon of Himalayan salt to fairly warm soaking water to trigger the enzymes that deactivate the enzyme inhibitors. Cover with water one inch above the nuts and seeds. Each time you pour off the water and refresh with more warm water, add another teaspoon of Himalayan salt. Change the water one to two times. If the nuts swell, the water level will also drop and will need to be topped off.

After soaking for twelve to eighteen hours, drain off the water, spread out flat on a baking sheet, and dry in an oven at 115°F for twelve to eighteen hours, or until the nuts are dried all the way through. You may also use a dehydrator for drying. Dehydrated nuts can be kept for up to twelve weeks in the refrigerator.

Note: cashews are already soaked before the shells are removed, so you do not need to soak them longer than one to two hours, or they may become slimy.

GRAINS (INCLUDING RICE)

The complex antinutrients in grains and rice contain require lemon juice or baking soda to aid in deactivating them. We recommend adding one teaspoon of baking soda or lemon juice to grains that are covered with about one inch of warm water. Soak them for twelve to twenty-four hours, changing the water once or twice. Don't forget to replenish the lemon juice or baking soda each time you change the water, and keep them covered about one inch above the grains throughout the process. You will need to keep a close eye on rice, as it absorbs more water than any other grain.

When you are done soaking, rinse the grains, pour them into your cooking pan and cook in fresh water until al dente. Be careful not to overcook your grains. They should not be overly soft. If you plan to store the grains, spread them flat on a baking sheet and dehydrate in the oven until completely dry. Use only sprouted, dehydrated grains and beans to process into flours in the Vitamix. And only make enough flour to use at a time for optimal freshness and nutritional content. It will make a difference in the taste of your baked items.

Wheat is one of the grains we don't even consider eating because of the genetic manipulation that has happened over many years through hybridization and backcrossing. Dr. William Davis wrote about this in detail in *Wheat Belly*. Einkorn, which is grown from heritage seed, is the exception.

Seventeen

PANTRY STAPLES TO HAVE ON HAND

BETH AND EDDIE

When starting to cook most of your meals from scratch, there can be some items you may want to keep on hand at all times to make it easier on your production schedule.

Some of the most important pantry staples are dried herbs and seasoning mixes. We have included some seasoning mix recipes in our cookbook to help you in this regard. There will be times when you will want to limit the type of dried herbs you use, especially when you are in Phases 1 and 2 of the Misner Plan. During Phase 3, unless you continue to have an inflammatory response in your body (some signs are painful joints, swelling, allergies, skin irritation, and/or congestion), most all dried herbs are fine to use. If this is true for you, stay with the Phase 2 herbs we recommend.

The dried herbs we keep in our kitchens are as follows:

- Basil
- Bay leaves
- Cayenne and red pepper flakes
- Cilantro
- Cinnamon (powdered and sticks)
- Cumin

- Dill
- Fennel
- Garlic, powdered
- Ginger
- Herbes de Provence
- Lemon zest, oven dried
- Italian seasoning
- Mustard, dry rubbed
- Onion, powdered
- Oregano
- Parsley
- Peppercorns (red, green, and black)
- Rosemary
- Sea salt
- Seaweed flakes (dulse, kelp, etc.)
- Thyme
- Turmeric
- Vanilla bean (both fresh and powdered)

The Misner Plan seasoning mixes we use the most and keep at the ready are below:

- Creole Seasoning Mix
- Dill Seasoning Mix
- Indonesian Seasoning Mix
- Southwestern Seasoning Mix

Sweeteners to keep on hand during Phase 3 (in order of preference)

- Apples for making applesauce
- Pears for making pear sauce
- Dates for making date puree
- Raw, local honey
- Raw, organic coconut nectar
- Raw, organic maguey sap
- Raw, organic agave

Eighteen

ANIMAL PROTEINS

BETH

When Ivan and I were considering how to eat in a way that best nourished our bodies during his healing phase, getting lean, clean sources of protein became very important. By clean, I mean easy for his body to break down and digest with little or no harmful chemicals or other substances for his liver to process out, such as saturated fats. We had to learn a lot about protein sources and why certain types of foods were harder to metabolize than others and stressed the liver or brought in substances that were toxic to the entire body.

Many people, including oncologists and nutritionists, advocate a vegetarian or vegan diet as the most healthful way to eat. We read quite a lot of the current research that shows how carcinogenic animal proteins can be when we were considering how we planned to proceed. There is no denying the conclusions of this research—animal proteins have a carcinogenic effect on the body.

We have noticed, as have others, that there is little specification in the research about how animal proteins are prepared. There doesn't seem to be any differentiation made between whether the animal proteins are sourced from industrialized factory farms (including farmed fish) or wild, free-range or pasture-raised, grass-fed or, in the case of eggs, cage-free. And I mean really cage-free, not just where the girls are given the option to go out into a small pen for an hour per day, which the hens may or, as is more probable, may not do.

Could it be that the industrialization of today's factory farms is what has made eating the foods we have eaten for centuries without all these side effects so detrimental today? In other words, when eaten in moderation, grass-fed or wild meats, pasture-raised eggs, and wild-caught fish (the smaller fish known to be lower in mercury toxicity), we believe, can be a healthy part of our diet.

The Omnivore's Dilemma by Michael Pollan provides a lot to consider when deciding what kind of animal protein to eat. Most of us don't even think twice about this. We just go to the market and purchase whatever either looks good or is on sale. Or maybe we are buying our animal protein from one of the bulk stores that are bringing in meats from other countries with questionable regulations.

Most people don't stop to consider the source of the meats, fish, and eggs we eat, much less how these creatures are being mistreated. There is a sobering YouTube video that allows you to actually see inside the factory farms and witness the unnatural conditions the cows, pigs, and chickens are subjected to.

Pollen also illuminates these aspects of farming in his book. He goes deeply into how our industrialized, factory-farmed animals are being fed, which is a huge part of the equation, not to mention the antibiotics and growth hormones they are pumped full of. After reading his book, we realized that if the animals we eat for food can no longer even sustain their own lives beyond just a few years, why should we be surprised that we are also damaged by what is damaging them when *we eat them*?

After going deep into the research and dynamics of how animal proteins affect our bodies, we have realized that it is possible, even desirable, to eat the right kinds of meats, eggs, and fish prepared properly to maximize their benefit and minimize their potential to damage our health. Animal protein has all the amino acids our bodies need to thrive. Amino acids are vital to good brain function and muscle development, and they enhance our immune systems.

You may know that we don't produce all the amino acids we need for health. Yes, it is possible to be healthy on a vegetarian or a vegan diet, getting all the amino acids by including a wide variety of vegetable protein sources to be sure we are covered. We believe it is possible to be healthy on a regular diet that includes small amounts of animal proteins, too. It takes knowledge and planning to do either.

We decided to include lean, clean sources of animal protein in the Misner Plan. I can tell you that we have radically reduced the amount of animal protein in our diet from before Ivan's diagnosis. We no longer have meat at all three meals. We typically will have egg whites with a heated but uncooked yolk for breakfast (we'll explain why), meat or fish for lunch, and then we have a vegetarian meal for supper.

One of the first animal protein sources added back in after Phase 1 is eggs. We used to think buying organic eggs at the local grocery store chain was adequate, even preferable. Then we learned a lot more about eggs. When possible, we buy eggs from a local farmer who brings them to the farmers' market. We know this farmer, and we were able to ask him if he's feeding his hens GMO grains or not (he's not and was insulted when we even asked). When that is not possible, we buy pasture-raised, non-soy-fed, organic eggs from another trust-worthy source. To find out where you can buy pasture-raised eggs, check www.eatwild.com.

Of special note: If you can get eggs that come from chickens being fed a non-GMO diet, celebrate! Most "vegetarian" chicken feed will include GMO grains, such as soy.

The term "cage-free eggs" has little or no meaning of significance. The hens can still be crowded in the factory farm's barn with very little room, and they are not eating what normal, healthy chickens need to eat to stay healthy or to produce healthy eggs. When we learned what the US Department of Agriculture (USDA) considers to be cage-free, I laughed. Then I immediately felt bad. The poor chickens. If you want to know more about the various designations and what they actually mean, visit www.humanesociety.org. Our local farmer at Coyote Creek Farms in Elgin, Texas, said, "As soon as we can get the chicks out of the barn, the better they do." I actually stopped to write that gem down.

We also learned a little bit more about how eggs are processed and brought to market in the United States. After being removed from the cages, the eggs must be washed and sanitized, as mandated by the USDA. This washing and sanitization removes the natural protective layer of the egg, or cuticle, which is perfectly designed to protect the egg from bacterial contamination.

You see, eggshells are porous, and the cuticle seals the eggs so that they are less likely to absorb bacteria after having been lain. While the USDA classifies egg washing and destaining compounds as potential food additives because they may be absorbed into the egg itself, the FDA has no published regulations for the egg producers to follow. Some states even require that the eggs be coated with vegetable or mineral oil, a petroleum product, before being sold. If you've ever had trouble getting egg whites to form peaks when beaten, you may be in one of these states.

In the European Union, it is illegal to wash the eggs at all before selling them. The reasoning is there is more risk of contamination when the cuticle is stripped away by our fervent washing. And truly, you are not going to be ridding the eggs of all possible salmonella by fervent washing and sterilization since the bacteria are harbored in the hen's reproductive tract and can actually be inside the egg, not only on the shells. US hens are not typically immunized against salmonella—EU hens are.

Larger organic farms usually use a nontoxic, organic, USDA-approved wash and sterilization solution. If the farm has less than three thousand hens, it is not held to these regulations. These farms may dry brush their eggs or use a gentle washing method that does not compromise the cuticle. This is another reason to frequent your local farmers' market and to make friends with that neighbor or coworker who has chickens. You might even consider setting up your own backyard chicken coop if your zoning laws will allow it. One of my Texas friends whose HOA prohibits chickens was able to have quails, whose eggs offer superior nutrition compared to chicken eggs.

Egg whites are a very clean source of protein. They are easy for us to metabolize, and they are fat-free and low in calories. There are no rules about how to prepare them. We feel that unless you are buying your eggs from a reliable source, you should cook them and not eat them raw because of the potential to be exposed to salmonella. Another reason for cooking egg whites is that they contain biotin, a B vitamin we need, but they are also high in avidin, which binds the biotin and keeps it from being metabolized in our bodies. Heating the egg deactivates the avidin and releases the biotin so we can assimilate it.

There are a few important things to know about egg yolks. The dietary cholesterol eggs are known for is contained in the yolk. While dietary cholesterol is not something to be concerned about with Misner Plan foods, if you have high cholesterol, you will not want to be eating two or three yolks per day. We do not eat more than five yolks each per week. When Ivan had active cancer in the prostate, he did not eat egg yolks at all. They are high in omega-6 fat or arachidonic acid (AA). If there is any inflammatory condition present in the body, levels of AA can be problematic, because AA is a proinflammatory fatty acid.

Another reason to not cook the egg yolk is that the omega-6 fat becomes damaged when subjected to heat long enough or high enough to cook it. The omega-6 fat in eggs cannot stand up to very much heat at all. Remember the point about biotin and avidin? It applies to the yolk, too.

We eat soft-boiled or poached eggs with the yolks still runny. Cooked this way, the avidin is deactivated, and the biotin is released to be metabolized by the body. We also eat scrambled egg whites and gently set one egg yolk in the middle of each portion before taking the pan off the heat source so that it will be heated enough to deactivate the avidin. If you will be using a raw egg in a smoothie or Orange Julius, deactivate the avidin by holding the egg with tongs under hot running water for about sixty seconds before breaking into the blender. We do bake with eggs when needed in a recipe, and if a flax egg can be substituted (such as in a bread, muffin, or pancake recipe), you may opt use it instead.

To make a flax egg, grind fresh, organic sprouted flaxseeds in a coffee grinder reserved for processing herbs. Mix one tablespoon flax meal immediately with three tablespoons water and refrigerate until set, about fifteen minutes.

Many people ask us what we think about following the Paleo eating protocol. It's a complicated answer. There are many great things about going Paleo: eliminating dairy, sugars, gluten grains, and processed foods. There is, in our opinion, too much emphasis on animal proteins. We are glad for the awareness eating Paleo is bringing to its followers regarding what kind of meat they eat. Grass-fed beef is part of a Paleo menu. There is a good reason why grass-fed beef is superior to corn-fed beef.

Quite simply, Cows are not able to digest grains properly. Their digestive systems are not designed to metabolize grains. They are grazing ruminates and need grasses in order to be healthy. When they are fed corn, oats, and other grains, their bodies produce toxins—too many to be eliminated by the animals. They store these toxins in their flesh, usually in their fat cells, just like we do. Because of the contents of their diets, the fat in industrially raised, factory-farmed cows is not the healthy omega-3 fat. They are the omega-6 fats most of us are typically getting too much of. Then to top it off, we cook the meat, which creates harmful free radicals and damages the fats.

When you add the use of antibiotics to keep the animals alive long enough to get them from hoof to plate to this already less-than-optimal situation, as well as the growth hormones used to accelerate this process and increase profits, the resulting food product is not on the Misner Plan.

Wild meats such as buffalo, elk, venison, and ostrich are all fine on the Misner Plan, as are goat and lamb. Again, you need to know your ranches when you purchase these meats, since some bison and elk are beginning to be factory farmed, too. Natural bison given a "vegetarian diet" is a fancy marketing tactic. Hold out for grass-fed, grass-finished!

Our guideline for personal health is to have red meat no more than once every two weeks. We typically do not eat these meats at restaurants, unless we can be sure they are truly wild meats.

Pork is not on the food list for the Misner Plan. You may wonder why that is. Pork growers want us to think of their product as "the other white meat," which has become associated with higher levels of health and desirability. But the reason pork is white, not pink, does not make it desirable at all!

Basically, pigs are lazy! They do not have the same kind of blood flow to their tissue as cows, sheep, or goats. The oxygen-storing compound, myoglobin, is in short supply for these large, typically overly fat mammals. Their flesh is also much higher in cholesterol and satu-rated fat than cows, sheep, or goats.

Most pork products are also preserved with nitrates and nitrites and are full of sugars, such as high-fructose corn syrup and maple syrups, and include smoke flavors, all of which are not useful for detoxing the body or maintaining health. Nitrates and nitrites have also been implicated as cancer-causing agents. As such, we avoid pork products on the Misner Plan.

Going wild with respect to meat relates to seafood, too. The introduction and proliferation of farmed fish has its drawbacks. Because the fish are held in closer-than-normal quarters, their environment becomes more and more polluted with their own waste by-products.

Much like their four-legged counterparts in factory farms, disease becomes more problematic, so they are given antibiotics they do not receive in the wild. It is nearly impossible to find tilapia in the store that is not farmed. We do not use tilapia in any of our recipes. We do not eat it at all. Farmed salmon can often have red dye added to it, which is another chemical we do not want to ingest.

Another issue with fish is the toxic levels of the ocean waters where they are swimming. Here is a good rule of thumb—the smaller the fish, the fewer toxins it is likely to have. Medium-size fish eat the smaller fish, larger fish eat the medium-size fish, and the giants of the seas eat everything smaller than themselves. You can see how the toxic burden of the fish increases with their size. The fish we have removed from our menus includes tuna, Chilean sea bass, shark, swordfish, and marlin.

King mackerel and orange roughy are also high on the mercury-toxicity list but are not commonly on restaurant menus or at our stores' fish counters.

The Department of Health and Human Services (HHS), the Environmental Protection Agency (EPA), and the Food and Drug Administration (FDA) keep track of the various fish and their levels of mercury. Below is an outline from the FDA's website report of the most well-known fish for you to take a peek at. Note: the most recent data is from 2014, so check with your local state agencies for more updated information. The data does not specify if the fish are wild-caught or farmed. The only designation is "commercially fished."

Fish species (uncooked) and parts per million of methylmercury detected (arranged from highest to lowest):

Shark	0.988
Swordfish	0.976
King mackerel	0.730
Orange roughy	0.554
Marlin	0.485
Bass, Chilean	0.386
Tuna, canned	0.353
Lobster	0.310
Halibut	0.252

Snapper	0.189
Monkfish	0.180
Perch	0.140
Trout	0.072
Cod	0.095
Crab	0.060
Catfish	0.049
Pollock	0.041
Anchovy	0.043
Haddock	0.031
Sardine	0.016
Salmon	0.014
Oyster	0.013
Shrimp	Undetectable

When eating fish on the Misner Plan, we try to have a side serving of freshly chopped cilantro with it. Cilantro is highly regarded for its escort ability to keep mercury moving through the digestive system until it is eliminated. Drinking cilantro juice shots when eating fish regularly could also be helpful. Strawberries are also known to play the role of escort for mercury contained in fish.

Nineteen

From Farm to Table

Beth

"Farm to table" has become a popular phrase added to marketing pieces for many food markets, menus in gourmet restaurants serving artisan foods, and subtitles of fancy cookbooks. But what does it really mean? And is it important in the Misner Plan?

I was recently shopping in a local health-oriented market when I saw a large, full-color poster of a woman holding a chicken. The caption was "Know where your food comes from." I guess the implication was that she knew the farm that the chicken was living on before she bought it all neatly wrapped up in plastic in the store and took it home to cook for dinner. But I think we are all clear that this is a marketing ploy. You don't really know where your food is coming from when you buy it from one of these markets.

And maybe you've seen the viral video of the cows, pigs, and chickens being processed in one of the factory packaging centers somewhere in Asia. I had a hard time bringing myself to watch that video, but I made myself do it. Watching that video helped me break some bad buying habits I had slipped into. But more about that later.

The truth is that you will not know about the food you are eating when you buy it at the store unless you can buy something labeled with a farm's name that you personally know and whose farming practices you are familiar with.

This is the main reason Ivan and I try to do most of our shopping at our local farmers' market. It's another part of the reason we moved to Austin, Texas, at the end of 2013. If you are fortunate enough to live in a community where you have access to real farms and real farmers, not industrial farms or land covered up by cement, you can visit these farms, and even pick your own organic produce in many cases. Or you might be able to help with the capture and butchering of your evening meal's chicken dish. Although I have not participated in any of the latter activities, I have been able to get to know the Smith family, from whom I buy eggs and chicken, and the folks at Boggy Creek Farm where I get farm-fresh produce that is not grown with chemical fertilizers or any pesticides at all.

One Saturday morning at my local farmers' market, I asked Farmer Bill if his tomatoes were certified organic. This was his prickly reply: "I don't need a government agency giving me a certification for my organic crops. I don't use pesticides. Never have, never will." And he took umbrage at my question, I can assure you.

But why has farm to table become so desirable that even huge, corporate markets are using it in their advertising campaigns?

So much research has been done, and studies have shown that food begins to lose its nutritional value as soon as it is harvested. Here is a short science lesson for you in everyday English. When plants are attached to the source and are growing, taking in air and water, producing the phytochemicals that interact so powerfully and positively with our body systems, there are vast reserves of antioxidants coursing through their stems, leaves, flowers, and fruits. As soon as they are harvested, they continue to "breathe," but they are no longer connected to the source in a kind of closed circuit to prevent moisture loss and oxidation.

An enzymatic process begins, and the plant starts to decay and oxidize as soon as it is removed from the growing medium. Nutritional levels begin dropping as respiration continues. In some plants this drop happens much more quickly than in others. All plants that are high in water-soluble vitamins, such as the B-complex vitamins and vitamin C, begin to lose their vitamin potency quickly.

When you buy produce from the store, you can bet it was picked days, sometimes weeks ago. The rule of thumb we follow with the Misner Plan is to eat fruits within two to three days of being picked and vegetables within three to five days.

There is so much to be said about how processing food reduces the nutritional values, so we will leave it at this: the most effective way to preserve the nutritional values of fresh fruits and vegetables if you aren't going to be eating them within the first few days you bring them home is to buy them as freshly picked as possible from your farmers' market; wash them well; then chop, blanch, and freeze in BPA-free plastic or glass freezer containers. That way you can use them over a week or two without losing too much of the nutritional value.

The second-best way to eat fruits and vegetables, if you are not able to buy them from the farmers' market and eat or freeze right away, is to buy frozen organics. These fruits and vegetables are usually processed quite close to the farms, and the length of time they continue to breathe is shorter than what you are going to have access to "fresh" in your regular stores. A quick Google search will reveal that some of the produce in the stores was harvested weeks or months previously and kept in cold storage after being chemically treated.

In all our recipes, we recommend organic vegetables. It is important to understand that the label Certified Organic does *not* mean no pesticides or chemicals were used to produce the food. It varies from state to state, but there is a wide variety of chemical sprays and powders permitted on organic crops. For this reason it is very important to wash the produce in a way that will denature whatever chemical residues may be on the skin or peels of your produce.

Soak the produce in a large bowl of purified water with one cup of white vinegar. Drain the water/vinegar mixture after three minutes and lightly scrub, then rinse the produce. Now soak the produce in purified water with two tablespoons of baking soda dissolved in it. Drain the water/baking soda mixture after three minutes and scrub the produce thoroughly under fresh, running water. This method will remove chemical residues and kill any bacteria on the peels.

It is important to clean the peels of all your produce before preparing and eating, even the foods from which you normally remove the peel or outer layers, such as onions, garlic, spaghetti squash, oranges, lemons, and avocados. Cutting through the unwashed peels can transfer chemical residue to the interior of the fruit or vegetable and further contaminate the produce.

The fruits and vegetables that are likely to be the least contaminated by pesticides when conventionally grown are:

Asparagus
Avocados
Cabbage
Cantaloupe
Corn
Eggplant
Grapefruit
Kiwi
Mangoes
Mushrooms
Onions
Papayas
Pineapples
Sweet potatoes

The fruits and vegetables that are likely to be the MOST contaminated by pesticides when conventionally grown (these should be avoided unless you can get organically grown) are:

Apples
Celery
Cherry tomatoes
Cucumbers
Grapes
Hot peppers
Nectarines
Peaches
Potatoes
Spinach
Strawberries
Sweet bell peppers
Kale
Zucchini squash

Regarding genetically engineered fruits and vegetables, there are quite a few in our grocery store produce sections, which are GMO. The best way to be sure to avoid them is to purchase only the organically grown varieties. Certified organic fruits and vegetables are not genetically modified.

The produce most likely to be GMO when conventionally grown are:

Corn
Green peas
Papaya
Potatoes
Soybeans/edamame
Tomatoes
Yellow squash
Zucchini squash

There are a lot of people writing and teaching about the importance of eating seasonal foods that are grown in your locality. The concept here is that our body chemistries allow for premium digestion and metabolizing of the nutrients from our own environment, rather than foods that are more exotic and/or are out of season in our geographic region.

While Ivan and I did not closely adhere to this practice during Ivan's healing season, it does seem to make sense to us overall, and we are moving closer to the ideal of eating foods grown in our area in their respective growing seasons from the simple result of shopping at the local farmers market. There is research available which shows our bodies respond specifically to fruits higher in carbohydrates that are ripe and typically ready to be harvested in the late summer by allowing us to store energy (in the form of fat), which prepares our bodies for the winter season. This process is described thoroughly in Dr. Steven R. Grundy's book, *Diet Evolution: Turn Off the Genes That Are Killing You—And Your Waistline—And Drop the Weight for Good* and is the basis for Eric Edmeades's WildFit program. Since Ivan and I are eating more from our local farms, as I mentioned, this is naturally happening with our meals. It is a different story when we travel.

An aspect of the "eating foods grown in your region" practice that we adhere to quite closely has to do with the types of fats we consume. Omega-6 fats are high in plant sources grown at the equator. As we humans live farther away from the equatorial center of the earth, our bodies' need for omega-6 fats is reduced, and we need a different ratio of fats in our diets.

This is very important when it comes to the types of nuts and oils we eat, especially during a healing phase where you might want to reduce the levels of arachidonic acids (omega-6 fats) being consumed in order to reduce their proinflammatory effect in your body.

Dr. Udo Erasmus has written what most nutritionists view as the bible on fats. We highly recommend his book *Fats That Heal, Fats That Kill: The Complete Guide to Fats, Oils, Cholesterol and Human Health.* This book is technical, but it also has easy-to-understand sections that will help you with this balancing act. For a book that anyone can easily understand, we recommend Dr. Mark Hyman's book *Eat Fat, Get Thin.*

Twenty

Too Sweet to Eat

BETH

The Misner Plan's success in building up a strong immune system lies with its ability to reprogram our taste buds. Most of us gravitate toward sweet tastes, and there is a very good reason for this. Eric Edmeades shared with us that before humans had access to industrialized, processed foods, sweet meant more energy, more antioxidants, and more calories. Think for a moment about when it is that most all brightly-colored fruits, in particular, are at their ripest. They are incredibly sweet.

Even our high-carbohydrate vegetables, the ones that are the sweetest, are usually brightly colored and high in antioxidants. Think again about deep-orange carrots; bright-orange, yellow, and purple sweet potatoes; red, yellow, and orange bell peppers; red, yellow, and green tomatoes; bright-green peas; and deep-yellow sweet corn. Your taste buds come alive, and perhaps you begin to salivate just reading about them. They are high in energy—energy in the form of simple carbohydrates.

In his book *Dr. Grundy's Diet Evolution*, Dr. Grundy explains quite well how this dynamic worked for our ancestors and why it is harming us today. His conclusion is that we have constant access to high-fructose foods and have even created new high-fructose ingredients that contribute to this energy-storing factor when we don't need it. The overexposure to high-fructose ingredients is wreaking havoc with our blood glucose levels and causing many of the illnesses we face today.

Dr. Hyman expounds even further on the dangers of a high-sugar diet, which most of us naturally gravitate toward and which our industrialized food stream has been so brilliant at creating for us. In his many books about the "blood sugar solution," he addresses the chemical mechanics of why eating too many high-sugar foods (including too much fruit and predominantly the high-sugar vegetables) is not optimal for our health. The Misner Plan starts out with removing most sugars from the diet for a time to allow detoxification and balance to be realized. That is why we eliminate fruits, except lemons, and all the sweet vegetables.

To be sure, you cannot have life without sugars. Glucose is what gives cells their energy to perform their intricate functions and keep us alive. Nearly everything we eat is broken down so thoroughly that the basic components are released. Glucose is one of those components.

During Phase 1 of the Misner Plan, you still get sugars, but they will come from low-carbohydrate vegetables and complex-carbohydrate grains that have been prepared in such a way that your body can utilize the sugars for building up your health rather than allowing them to contribute to the breakdown of your health. It has a lot to do with the very complicated dance the body does with insulin production and the metabolization of sugars.

Another reason the Misner Plan reduces sugar intake at the onset is to help you regain the proper balance of beneficial bacteria as compared to yeasts and other fungi that contribute to your body's toxic burden. When we eat the standard American diet, we are actually feeding the bad guys who thrive on sugars, and we do not support the good guys who are critical to our health.

Biochemists estimate that each of us carries approximately 3 percent of our body's weight in microbes. In terms of measuring the total number of cells in the body, the microbes themselves outnumber our human cells by ten to one, or more than ten thousand microbial species, according to the National Institutes of Health (NIH) website. There is literally more nonhuman DNA in our bodies than human DNA. And we have to know how to keep the balance right, or we can become sick.

The colonies of beneficial bacteria that live in our small intestines play an extremely necessary role in food digestion and the metabolizing of nutrients. They break down the macronutrients (fat, carbs, and proteins) into substances we can absorb. They also produce enzymes, vitamins, and anti-inflammatory substances we don't make for ourselves. We need these co-laborers. Our bodies' digestive processes are incomplete without them, and our health suffers.

The proliferation of antibiotic use is often pointed to as the primary cause of dysbiosis. Coupled with a diet that does not create an environment that is hospitable to our beneficial bateria's life cycle, you get a one-two knockout punch that has an adverse effect on our lives.

The beneficial bacteria depend on an alkaline environment to live and work to keep us healthy. When our diets are predominantly acidic, we create an environment in our guts that promotes the growth of microbes that do not help us with digestion (opportunistic microbes/bacteria) and actually harm the colonies of beneficial bacteria. We then start to experience nutritional deficiencies. We begin to experience the toxic side effects from the opportunistic microbes that thrive in a state of dysbiosis in our guts.

Dysbiosis is the scientific way of referring to an imbalance in the gut flora that tips the scale in the opportunistic microbes' favor. It was interesting for us to learn that the food we eat is critical for avoiding dysbiosis and remaining in homeostasis, the condition of the body when all the systems are balanced and working well. The opportunistic microbes excrete substances like methane gasses (are you feeling bloated?—that could be why), while the beneficial bacteria excrete hydrogen peroxide that actually keeps the opportunistic microbes from multiplying. It is a factor of our kitchen practices that we really try to pay attention to now that we are more aware of the many important reasons to do so.

Sugar feeds these opportunistic microbes faster than anything else. Sugar also feeds yeast and other microorganisms that can actually suppress our immune systems. An overabundance of yeast in our digestive system can lead to fermentation in our guts. You know you are fermenting in the gut if you develop gas after eating something that is known to feed yeasts.

Picture bread dough rising as a result of the fermentation happening with the yeast feeding on the sugars in the dough. Do you ever feel like your belly is rising just like that dough? If you do, then you can be pretty sure you are fermenting after you eat.

So what are we to do?

First of all, after completing the cleanse in Phase 1 of the Misner Plan, you will want to use complex-carbohydrate sweeteners and eliminate processed, simple sugars. Notice I did not say eliminate sugar, but rather "processed sugar." Remember that we need sugar to survive, but we need our bodies to work at producing glucose; we do not want to dump it in the hopper, ready to go. Processed sugar and other simple carbohydrates can also cause a rapid spike in insulin, which can lead to damage to our cells' ability ultimately to absorb glucose. This is the primary factor in the onset of type 2 diabetes.

Once you have completed Phase 1, you will be adding back in some dairy products (goat's or sheep's milk yogurt and cheeses), and dairy contains more sugars than you have been eating during the 8-Day Detox. The key is to go slowly. Don't start immediately pigging out on dairy products. Just have a little bit now and then.

At the end of Phase 1, our bodies have just begun the toxic release process. During Phase 2, we are still releasing, and our overall body chemistry fluctuates as it moves toward the optimal condition. It is in Phase 2, depending on the individual's quantity of toxic buildup and release, that you may begin to settle in the normal pH range. It is wise to stay in Phase 2 until you see a steady pH reading as you continue to check your urine pH.

When you are in Phase 3, keep an eye on your body's cues to learn when you may need to pull back from using the natural, complex-carbohydrate sweeteners permitted on the Misner Plan and when you may need to even slow down on fruit and the higher-carb veggies. It can be helpful to move into a three-day cleanse if you start to recognize the signs of dysbiosis (bloating, gas, change in stool pattern, urine pH readings that are getting higher or more alkaline) in order to give your beneficial bacteria a boost in their bid for real estate in your gut. We need to learn to eat to cultivate these colonies, since they are so vital to our own health.

After Phase 2, you will be able to add back in the sweeter veggies and fruits. At this time you can also begin using some natural, complex-carbohydrate sweeteners for baking.

We like to use sweeteners in this order:

Fruit puree (applesauce, pear sauce, mashed bananas, and date puree)
Local wild, raw honey

Raw maguey sweet sap
Raw coconut nectar
Date sugar
Coconut sugar
Raw agave

Once in Phase 3, if fluctuating pH levels occur, it would be wise to settle back into Phase 2 and monitor and reduce the amounts and combinations of grain, oil, fruits, and higher carbohydrate vegetables, as well as the recommended natural sweeteners. Use the carbohydrate content chart to guide you in moving back to lower-carb fruits and vegetables.

Grains can create dysbiosis in the gut, too. Even eating sprouted grain flours can give opportunistic bacteria quicker access to glucose, and that can lead to their proliferation. We try to have baked goods or use any of the recipes with flours no more than two or three times per week. Fourless (or Paleo) breads, muffins, or pancakes are better options. Before the Misner Plan, we were eating something with some kind of flour in it at nearly every meal! Think about your diet for a moment. Are you eating that way now, too?

When we were new to this way of thinking about food, agave was a very attractive choice. Touted as low glycemic, it seemed to be a great alternative to sugar, even better than honey. As we have moved deeper into this plan, we have learned a couple of things about agave that have relegated it to the once-in-a-while category, and then used only when labeled raw.

Syrup and molasses are processed by their very natures. They must be boiled in order to concentrate the sweetness of the sap/juice. In the case of regular agave, the high-heat processing it undergoes creates an extremely high-fructose sweetener, which is not desirable at all. Raw agave may be processed at a temperature under 118°F, which keeps it on the Misner Plan's approved list. However, just looking at a label in the grocery store will not tell you if that manufacturer kept the temp under 118°F or not. This is why it is *last* on the list, and why we caution you to know your source. Any recipe containing raw agave will be fine if you substitute maguey sap, discussed next.

Since Ivan's healing experience, we have learned about another sweetener that comes from the agave plant: maguey sap. This sweet juice comes from the stalk of the agave plant, while agave syrup is produced by processing the roots of the plant. Both maguey sap and coconut nectar do not need to be boiled in order to concentrate their sweetness. Coconut nectar comes from the naturally sweet sap of the coconut palm (not the same palm from which we derive palm oil) and is typically dehydrated, not boiled.

Maguey sap and raw coconut nectar are enzymatically "alive," which means they are not being heated above 118°F, and they do not have the high-fructose content of regular agave syrup. They are usually dehydrated. In the case of Villa de Patos's brand raw maguey, the temperature it is dehydrated at is no higher than 75°F. These sweeteners also contain high levels of minerals, vitamins, and amino acids, which is why we have included them. Maguey sap even has substantial fiber content and is quite alkaline. Both maguey sap and raw coconut nectar are minimally processed and unrefined.

Even better than these saps are simple, raw fruit purees made fresh at home in your Vitamix or blender. They contain the lower level of sweetness you may be looking for in Phase 3 and all the enzymes, fiber, and water of the whole fruit. They are always our first choice.

Points to ponder:

- Keep an eye on your urine pH. If it starts to quickly move too high, above the optimal range between 6.2 and 7.4, consider that you might be experiencing fermentation in the gut. Slow down on your intake of sweet foods, grains, and sweeteners. If it moves high and then drops low, you might be experiencing the production of vinegars in the gut, which is a part of the fermentation process and can cause your urine pH to become too acidic.
- Pay attention to any bloating or gas you may be experiencing. This can also indicate fermentation in the gut, and you will want to reduce sweets.
- Eat primarily low-carb veggies; soaked, cooked grains; and limited amounts of fruit.

Part Three

RECIPES

Twenty-One

PANTRY RECIPES

BETH AND EDDIE

These recipes have been created by Beth and Chef Eddie (and a couple of guest chefs making special appearances) specifically for the Misner Plan's three phases. As you take a stroll through our recipes, you will be able to quickly identify which chef created which recipes. Beth is a housewife, mother, and certified nutritionist. Her recipes are basic, yummy, and usually not very complicated. Adding to that and punching it waaaaay up is Chef Eddie, an executive chef who has cooked for five past US presidents and First Lady, Michelle Obama. Eddie is a native son of New Orleans. You will love his Cajun twist to the Misner Plan.

We have worked together to provide delicious, real-food recipes for you as you move between the three phases of the Misner Plan. Some of our recipes are actually ingredients in other, more complicated recipes. Where a recipe calls for ingredients that are created from other Misner Plan recipes, those ingredients will be listed as proper nouns, or uppercased.

To introduce our recipes, we share these points for you to keep in mind:

1. Use organically grown, carefully washed vegetables and fruits.
2. Fresh is always preferable, but where you cannot get fresh, frozen is an acceptable substitute.

3. Avoid GM ingredients. Corn, soy, canola, lecithin, or xanthan gum ingredients are all highly likely to be GM ingredients and are not included in the Misner Plan. If the product is 100 percent certified organic, you can be confident the ingredients are not GM.
4. Whenever water is called for in a recipe, use filtered or glass-bottled spring water if you do not have access to filtered tap water. Even cooking with unfiltered tap water will expose you to all the heavy metals and other toxins in the local water supply.
5. Avoid using yogurt and butter or ghee during Phases 2 and 3 if you have any type of inflammatory condition, including cancer, arthritis, an autoimmune disease, or the like. If you do not have any of these conditions, you may use small amounts of yogurt (preferably made from goat's or sheep's milk) and ghee made from organic butter from grass-fed cows during these two phases.
6. Any of the Phase 1 recipes may be used during Phase 2 and Phase 3. Any of the Phase 2 recipes may be used during Phase 3.
7. Regarding meats and fish called for in the recipes, always use hormone-free, antibiotic-free, pasture-raised or free-range, grass-fed, and grass-finished beef or bison, or wild-caught fish.
8. Use only the spices or spice mixes in our cookbook with phase-appropriate herbs during Phases 1 and 2, and use them liberally. They are packed with powerful phytonutrients, as well as antioxidants that have, in many cases, been the subject of medical research and have been found to contribute to healthy immune support.
9. Since cow dairy products are known to increase congestion and mucus production, they are eliminated in the Misner Plan, with the exception of cow's milk yogurt, which may be used only if you cannot obtain goat's or sheep's milk yogurt. We have some great ideas for milk alternatives in our book, so you won't even miss cow's milk. The occasional use of hard, dry-aged cow's milk cheeses, such as Asiago, Parmesan, and Pecorino Romano (traditionally made from sheep's milk in Italy, but made from cow's milk in the United States), is permitted during Phase 3, but in very small quantities. If you can get sheep-milk hard cheese, by all means, go with that.

A significant aspect of being able to succeed with the Misner Plan is to find fresh seasoning mixes, sauces, dressings, and dips you like. By substituting our recipes for processed, packaged, and chemically preserved items offered at the grocery store, you will experience a whole new world of flavors. The variety offered here emphasizes just how many choices you really do have on the Misner Plan.

Since we have arranged the pantry recipes alphabetically, we have indicated the phase each recipe fits in. Remember: Phase 1 recipes may be used in all three phases. Phase 2 recipes may be used in Phases 2 and 3. Phase 3 recipes may be used only in Phase 3. Some of the recipes have variations listed with them to show you how to adapt them to create variety and expand your repertoire.

Avocado Dressing

Chef Eddie
Yield: 6 servings
Phase 3

When I first started doing private aircraft catering, there was great emphasis on having variety, or different spins, on traditional dishes. Since I am a New Orleans guy, and we have great tomatoes we call Creole tomatoes, I was looking for a little twist on the famous Italian dish, Caprese. It's very difficult to beat the combination of a wonderfully ripe tomato, real mozzarella di Bufala, great extra-virgin olive oil, and a basil leaf. Classic and just plain good.

Well, I decided to add a slice of avocado, change the basil to cilantro, and then make an avocado-based dressing to go with it. It was a big hit and a top seller, and this dressing was a big reason. Score one for me that it is compatible with the Misner Plan.

Ingredients:
½ Haas avocado
½ jalapeño, seeded, stemmed, and diced
3 tablespoons red onion, chopped
½ cup cilantro, chopped
¼ cup lime juice, freshly squeezed
½ cup extra-virgin olive oil
1 tablespoon honey or maguey sap
Sea salt
Cayenne pepper

Instructions:
1. In a small food processor, Vitamix, or NutriBullet, combine all ingredients except olive oil and puree.

2. While the processor is running, stream in olive oil until you reach the desired consistency.

3. Give it a taste, adjust salt and pepper. It may need a little more lime juice to brighten it up. All of this varies with the size of the avocado and the flavor intensity of cilantro you start with. At the height of cilantro's freshness, you might find you actually need less lime juice.

Tip: If you're looking to reduce calories, put in half the oil and substitute the other half with Vegetable Stock. If the avocado is really fresh, ripe, and intense, you can skip the oil entirely if you like and just add stock.

Casablanca Rub

Chef Eddie
Yield: ¼ cup
Phase 3

Sometimes you just need to change the mood and go someplace different. This spice mixture does just that by combining the warm and spicy flavor profiles from cardamom, cumin, and coriander with seasonings that are more familiar and whisking you away to somewhere exotic.

Ingredients:
2 tablespoons spicy paprika
1 teaspoon coarse sea salt
¼ teaspoon ground ginger
⅛ teaspoon ground cardamom
2 teaspoons ground cumin
¼ teaspoon ground cloves
½ teaspoon cinnamon
½ teaspoon allspice
¼ teaspoon cayenne
½ teaspoon coriander

Instructions:
1. In small bowl, stir all ingredients.

2. Store in an airtight container.

Tip: this spice rub will keep at room temperature for up to 6 months.

Cashew Cream, Savory and Sweet

Chef Eddie
Yield: 2½ cups
Phase 3

When I was first asked to write this book and create great dishes from the Misner Plan food lists, I was a little concerned. Actually, I was scared! As I did research, I started to realize that there were some pretty good substitutes out there, and this is one of them. I have used cream sparingly in general and mostly as a flavor deepener or liaison, but this cream substitute will see more use in my kitchen, for sure. You can influence it with spice or sweet and can make it to the consistency you like. I love it.

Ingredients:

1 cup cashews, raw
½ to ¾ cup of filtered water (add more water according to consistency desired)

Instructions:

1. Place cashews in sealable container, add water to cover, and refrigerate overnight.

2. In the morning, place cashews and water into a Vitamix or some other mixer capable of pureeing (a blender or food processer will work if you don't have a Vitamix).

3. Gradually add more water and blend until the mixture is the consistency of heavy cream or whatever milk substitute you are trying to accomplish. You may have to strain the mixture through a fine-mesh screen or cheesecloth, depending on your blender. Use the prepared cream as soon as you make it so that no microorganisms have a chance to enjoy your cream before you do.

4. Finish the recipe by choosing one of the two variations below to complete the type of Cashew Cream you wish to make:

Savory Variation

Ingredients:
½ lemon, juiced
½ teaspoon sea salt
½ teaspoon apple cider vinegar, optional
1 clove garlic, optional
1 tablespoon extra-virgin olive oil, optional

Instructions:
Add ingredients to basic Cashew Cream and blend until smooth.

Sweet Variation
Ingredients:
2–4 tablespoons honey or maguey sap
¼ teaspoon powdered vanilla
¼ teaspoon cinnamon, optional

Instructions:
Add ingredients to basic cashew cream and blend until smooth.

Tip: The sweet variation makes a great pancake topping. It can also be drizzled over fruit and healthy desserts, like our Rhubarb Crumble. The savory cream can be used as a pizza topping, added to a healthy pasta dish, over vegetables, baked dishes, casseroles, healthy Mexican meals, as a salad dressing (it can be thinned down with additional olive oil), or wherever you may have added a savory, creamy sauce.

Creole Seasoning Mix

Chef Eddie
Yield: ¾ cup
Phase 3

This is a versatile seasoning mix, and you may find yourself using it in everything, even baby food—well, maybe not baby food, but I sauté nearly everything in it, mix it into my beans, season my soups, you name it. So, in my opinion, triple this recipe—it won't go to waste. Personally, I change every measurement to cups, as in 4 cups of paprika and 2 cups of sea salt. When I make a big batch, I give some away as gifts.

Ingredients:
4 tablespoons paprika
2 tablespoons sea salt
2 tablespoons garlic powder
1 tablespoon onion powder
¾ tablespoon cayenne pepper
1 tablespoon dried oregano
1 tablespoon dried basil
1 tablespoon dried thyme

Instructions:
1. Place all ingredients into a bowl and whisk together.

2. Transfer mix to an airtight jar.

Phase 2 Variation: omit paprika.

Creole Tartar Sauce

Chef Eddie
Yield: approximately 1¾ cups
Phase 3

This is a common seafood condiment in Louisiana, but it can also be used with sandwiches. And don't be afraid to experiment by using it wherever you would normally use mayo, like in egg salad.

Ingredients:

1 egg
1 tablespoon minced garlic
2 tablespoons lemon juice, freshly squeezed
1 tablespoon parsley leaves, chopped
2 tablespoons scallions, chopped
1 cup extra-virgin olive oil
¼ teaspoon cayenne pepper
1 teaspoon Vegan Worcestershire Sauce
1 tablespoon Creole or whole-grain mustard (made with apple cider vinegar)
1 teaspoon sea salt

Instructions:

1. Put egg, garlic, lemon juice, parsley, and scallions in a food processor and puree for 15 seconds.

2. With processor running, pour oil through the feed tube in a steady stream until mayonnaise forms.

3. Add cayenne, Vegan Worcestershire Sauce, mustard, and salt, and pulse once or twice to blend.

4. Cover and let sit for 1 hour in the refrigerator before using.

Dill Seasoning

Chef Eddie
Yield: ⅛ cup
Phase 1

Having good spice mixtures in your pantry is key, but many of the preblended, store-bought mixtures may have additives that are not included in the Misner Plan. Play with your spices and create flavors that accompany your personal flavor profile. Here is one to get you started. Remember, you don't have to make big quantities. Start with small batches (unless you are making my Creole Seasoning Mix, that is).

Ingredients:
1 tablespoon dried dill
1 teaspoon garlic powder
1 teaspoon onion powder
1 teaspoon horseradish root, ground and dried
1 teaspoon dried lemon zest
½ teaspoon sea salt
½ teaspoon cayenne pepper

Instructions:
1. Combine all ingredients together in a mixing bowl and toss with a spoon until well mixed.

2. Store in an airtight container.

Eddie's Caesar Dressing

Chef Eddie
Yield: 1 cup
Phase 3

Once you start making your own Caesar dressings, you will never consider a jarred version again. The zest, creaminess, and versatility of this make it a pantry must. Use as a dressing, dip, or spread. This varies from traditional Caesar Dressing since it does not contain anchovies, which some people do not like.

Ingredients:

2 egg yolks
2 tablespoons water or stock of your choice
1 tablespoon Dijon mustard, organic (make sure it's a brand free of sugar, such as Annie's)
½ cup Parmigiano Reggiano, grated
1 tablespoon lemon juice, freshly squeezed
1 clove garlic
½ cup extra-virgin olive oil
⅛ teaspoon salt, or to taste
⅛ teaspoon pepper

Instructions:

1. In food processor, combine egg yolks, water, Dijon mustard, Parmigiano Reggiano, lemon juice, and garlic.

2. Slowly add olive oil while blending constantly. Watch for the consistency to become very creamy.

3. Give it a taste as you go and adjust. I often find I have to add a little goat cheese or garlic to get it where I want because the quality of ingredients varies from time to time.

Tip: This is another dressing to use quickly. It will keep, jarred, for about 3 days.

Ghee

Chef Eddie
Yield: 2¼ cups
Phase 1

Don't let this intimidate you. It's pretty easy once you have done it, and the results are really worth it. Clarified butter smokes at a higher point, so sautéing with it is easier and adds a ton of flavor to whatever you're cooking. Use it to cook your scrambled eggs, cauliflower grits, and even add some to quinoa. It's incredible.

Ingredients:

1 pound butter, organic, grass-fed, unsalted

Equipment Needed:
Skillet with high sides
Fine-mesh skimmer
Fine-mesh strainer or cheesecloth
Glass container or Mason jar for storage

Instructions:

1. Heat a wide-bottomed skillet with high sides (to contain splashing/bubbling) over medium-low heat. Once warm, add butter. Use a wooden spoon or spatula to stir butter and speed along the melting process. It may take around 5 minutes.

2. Once the butter is completely melted and begins to bubble, slightly lower the heat. You want a steady bubble like a simmer, but not so much that butter is jumping out of the pan or splattering all over the stovetop. If that happens, lower the heat a tiny bit more. Cook until the milk protein has completely separated, and there is a layer on the top. There will be bits on the bottom of the pan as well, and you don't want those to burn.

3. Begin carefully skimming the top layer off until the ghee looks clean (except for bits on the very bottom) and discard. When you can see through to the bottom of the pan, the butter

has stopped bubbling, and you have skimmed off the top layer of foam, you are done. The butter should be clear and smell a little like caramel.

4. Once cool, strain through a fine-mesh strainer or cheesecloth. Discard the toasted bits from the bottom of the pan.

5. Store the ghee at room temperature in a glass container or Mason jar and use as needed.

Tip: mix with equal parts of olive oil to create a flavorful cooking oil.

Goat Cheese

Beth
Yield: 1 cup
Phase 3

Just in case you cannot find any goat cheese without mold inhibitors, I wanted to include a recipe so you could make your own goat cheese. You may like experimenting with this and simply make your own all the time just because it is fun, and you get an extreme sense of accomplishment, kind of like you would when making your own butter in order to make fresh ghee. This recipe produces a soft, mixable goat cheese perfect for creating herbed slathers to have with our homemade crackers and flatbreads.

Ingredients:

1 quart goat's milk (raw, if you can get it)
¼ cup lemon juice, freshly squeezed
½ clove garlic, freshly grated
3 pinches medium-ground sea salt or any other fresh herbs you would like to include

Instructions:

1. Heat goat's milk in a medium-size saucepan slowly to 180°F. Use a candy thermometer to check the temperature.

2. Once the milk reaches the desired temperature, remove from heat and stir in freshly squeezed lemon juice. Let the milk stand until it starts to curdle (about 20 minutes).

3. Set a colander inside a large bowl and line it with several layers of cheesecloth. If you do not use enough cheesecloth, the goat cheese can run through the colander into the bowl. Spoon milk into a cheesecloth-covered colander. Tie ends of cheesecloth around a wooden spoon laid across the colander so that it is lifted up from the surface of the colander to allow whey to drain off cheese. This may take up to 1½ hours.

4. When the cheese is the consistency of ricotta, gently transfer it from cheesecloth into a small bowl and stir in garlic, sea salt, and any other fresh herbs or dried fruit you would like to include.

Tip: gently stir in chopped chives, parsley, or rosemary.

Phase 3 Variation: add chopped, dried fruits, such as figs or sulfur-free dried apricots.

Grass-Fed Beef Bone Broth

Guest Chef Drew Saylor
Yield: approximately two quarts
Phase 3

Although I hated cooking as I grew up, I have worked in restaurants, kitchens, and around food my whole career. When I got my first job as a food expediter in a chain restaurant, I saw the chefs preparing meals for the guests every night and became fascinated with the precision and timing of everything. I started trying to make the things at home that I saw at work. After a few trials and errors, I learned how to make a few good meals, and I was hooked. I have become obsessed with ingredients, preparation, precision, timing, smells, and tastes. I have seen the importance of "real" food and how it can change your entire body's wellness. I first made this broth with the bones from a roast I made for my grandmother's birthday dinner. Cooking for your grandma is the real test of a chef, and I am happy to say I passed! This recipe is a must-have in my freezer during colder months to make stews, soups, casseroles, and stir-fry dishes.

Ingredients:
5 pounds grass-fed beef bones (from the roast cut, preferably with the marrow)
4 carrots, cut into 2- to 3-inch pieces
4 celery stalks, cut into 2- to 3-inch pieces
1 large leek, cut into 2- to 3-inch pieces
2 onions, cut into halves
1 head of garlic, cut in half
½ bunch flat-leaf parsley stems
4 sprigs thyme
4 bay leaves
1 tablespoon raw, unfiltered apple cider vinegar
2 tablespoons black peppercorns
12 cups filtered water

Instructions:

1. Preheat oven to 450°F. On a baking sheet, spread vegetable pieces. Place the bones on top of the vegetables and roast for 40 minutes. Toss everything after the first 20 minutes and place it back in oven until the vegetables are browned, about 20 more minutes.

2. Add the roasted bones and vegetables to a large stockpot, removing as much fat as possible before doing so. Add ½ cup of water to the baking sheet and scrape browned bits from the pan, adding them to the stockpot, as well. Pour in cold filtered water to cover by a few inches. Add thyme, parsley stems, bay leaves, peppercorn and vinegar to stockpot.

3. Bring to a boil, reduce heat, and simmer for 4-8 hours, up to 24! The longer it simmers, the more flavor you are extracting from all the ingredients. It is important to continually add water as necessary to keep everything covered by a few inches throughout the entire cook time. Skim fat off the top as often as possible while simmering.

4. Strain warm broth into a large bowl and pour it into quart jars for storage or use freshly made broth in your dish.

Tip: broth can be made 2 days ahead of time, if refrigerated, and will keep frozen for up to 3 months.

Herbed Orange Chèvre Slather

Beth
Yield: 1¾ cups
Phase 3

This slather makes a perfect topping for our Rosemary Walnut Crackers.

Ingredients:
8 ounces Goat Cheese
¼ cup yogurt, goat's or sheep's milk
Zest of medium orange
Pink, green, and black pepper, freshly ground
1 scallion, small dice
2 teaspoons fresh parsley, finely snipped

Instructions:
1. Mash Goat Cheese into yogurt in a medium-size bowl until combined.

2. Stir in orange zest and pepper.

3. With a rubber spatula, gently fold in scallions, and 1 teaspoon of parsley.

4. Spoon the mixture into a smaller bowl and garnish with remaining parsley. Refrigerate until ready to serve.

Homemade Baking Powder

Beth
Yield: 1 tablespoon
Phase 2

Since baking powder can often contain aluminum, it has become my practice to keep a jar of this mixed up and ready at all times in my pantry. When you realize how easy it is to make baking powder, you will be amazed. And you will probably never purchase store-bought baking powder again.

Ingredients:
1 teaspoon baking soda
2 teaspoons cream of tartar

Instructions:
1. Stir the baking soda and cream of tartar together until combined.

2. To store, add 1 teaspoon of non-GMO cornstarch to mixture (in order to absorb any moisture) and spoon the baking soda. Store tightly covered in a small jar.

Tip: to make more at one time, simply increase amounts of baking soda and cream of tartar, keeping the ratio 1:2.

Homemade Nut Butter

Beth
Yield: varies based on quantity of nuts used
Phase 3

Since the Misner Plan does not include peanuts on the food list, we have created a wide variety of nut butters. You will never miss peanut butter!

Ingredients:

2–4 cups of organic, soaked nuts, such as almonds, hazelnuts, cashews (may be dehydrated or lightly roasted)
1–2 tablespoons coconut oil
Sea salt, to taste (optional)

Instructions:

1. Pour the nuts into a food processor. Be sure there is room in the processor so that the nuts can swirl around freely.

2. Process on high until the nuts become powdered, between three to ten minutes, depending on what kinds of nuts you have chosen. At this point, you will need to scrape the sides of the bowl as you continue processing to the nut butter stage.

3. The mixture will turn creamy as it continues to swirl around in your processor. To assist with the process, add some of the coconut oil until you begin to see the consistency you prefer.

4. The salt can be added to your taste at the end of processing.

5. Transfer nut butter to a glass jar and refrigerate it to keep longer.

Tip: Your nut butter will process differently if you are using dehydrated nuts or lightly roasted nuts. The roasted nuts will take more oil to achieve the creamier texture you may want.

Horseradish Dill Dip

Chef Eddie
Yield: 1½ cups
Phase 3

This dip will make raw vegetables exciting and enjoyable to eat and cure any sinus ills you may have at the same time. The grated horseradish is the secret here. It absolutely sends this dip way over the top. Be careful to be downwind when grating it, and *don't* rub your eyes!

Ingredients:
½ cup yogurt, goat's or sheep's milk
½ cup lemon zest
½ cup fresh horseradish, grated
2 teaspoons fresh dill
Sea salt, to taste

Instructions:
1. Mix all ingredients in a bowl and refrigerate for 30 minutes to set.

2. Serve with vegetables.

Tip: will keep 7 days in the refrigerator.

Phase 2 Variation: serve with grilled or boiled shrimp. Make a Yogurt Dill Dip version of this recipe by doubling the yogurt and eliminating the horseradish.

Hummus

Chef Eddie
Yield: 1¼ cups
Phase 3

Hummus is a great all-around base for a wide variety of flavorful dips. I've given you a couple of variations to get you started. Now, you take it from here.

Basic Hummus

Ingredients:
1 cup chickpeas
⅓ cup extra-virgin olive oil
⅛ cup Vegetable Stock
2 teaspoons lemon juice, freshly squeezed
1 tablespoon Homemade Nut Butter, cashew
¼ teaspoon cayenne
Sea salt, to taste

Instructions:
1. In a small food processor, add prepared chickpeas, olive oil, Vegetable Stock, lemon juice, and Cashew Nut Butter. Combine until smooth.

2. Add salt and pepper to taste. Pulse to combine.

Red Pepper Hummus

Ingredients:
Hummus base
1 red pepper
Extra-virgin olive oil

Instructions:
1. Set the electric oven broiler to high and position the top rack 6–8 inches from the burner. Allow the broiler to heat.

2. Line a sheet pan with foil to protect the pepper from sticking. Place pepper on the sheet pan whole and brush the top with olive oil.

3. Broil the pepper for approximately 5 minutes, or until the skin is blackened.

Or:

1. Set the stovetop gas burner to a high flame.

2. Place the pepper directly on metal grate.

3. Turn the pepper with fire-safe tongs every 1–2 minutes until each side is blackened.

4. Once roasted, cool the pepper in a pot with the lid on. After 30 minutes, the charred skin will peel away.

5. Peel the skin off without rinsing under water, if you can. You are trying to retain oils from the pepper, and rinsing will cause them to be lost down the drain.

6. Remove the stems and seeds from the pepper and set aside.

7. In a small food processor, mix hummus and red pepper until combined.

8. Taste and adjust the seasoning.

Roasted Shallot Hummus

Ingredients:
¼ cup Basic Hummus
¾ cup Roasted Shallots

The sweetness of the shallots combined with the hummus makes this spread a sure winner. It's one you seldom see, so it's often the first one to disappear at parties. It also makes a great spread for a sandwich or tossed with a salad.

Instructions:
1. In a small food processor, puree the hummus and shallots until combined.

2. Taste and adjust seasonings, to taste.

Tip: enjoy hummus with Rosemary Walnut Crackers or with your favorite veggie sticks.

Indonesian Spice Mix

Chef Eddie
Yield: ¼ cup
Phase 1

This Phase 1-friendly blend gives a bit of a different flavor profile that more closely resembles what I have experienced in Indonesia, which makes it unique and interesting.

Ingredients:
1 tablespoon kosher salt
1 tablespoon dried cilantro
2 teaspoons dried basil
1 teaspoon dried parsley
1 teaspoon ground onion
1 teaspoon crushed red pepper
1 teaspoon Chinese five spice* (look for fennel seed, star anise, ginger, cloves, and cinnamon blends)
½ teaspoon ground garlic
½ teaspoon ground ginger
½ teaspoon ground coriander

Instructions:
1. Combine all ingredients in a mixing bowl and whisk until blended.

2. Store in an airtight container.

*There are many variations of the Chinese five-spice powder. You'll want to be sure it doesn't include black or white pepper in order to keep this seasoning mix in Phase 1.

Lemon Mint Dressing

Chef Eddie
Yield: 1¼ cup
Phase 1

Parsley gives this fresh dressing an herb-forward taste that pairs well with vegetables, chicken, and even some fish. This dressing will take some tasting and adjusting since there are many varieties of lemons and mint, but once you do it the first time, the next time will be a cinch.

Ingredients:

½ cup fresh mint leaves
⅓ cup extra-virgin olive oil
⅓ cup fresh lemon juice
1 teaspoon lemon zest, finely grated
1 small clove garlic (optional)
½ teaspoon sea salt
⅛ teaspoon cayenne
¼ teaspoon dry mustard
Honey or raw agave

Instructions:

1. Place ¼ cup of the lemon juice and all the other ingredients in a food processor and blend.

2. Give it a quick taste and adjust the seasonings. If the lemon isn't coming through, blend in the rest of it. If it's too tart, blend in a touch of honey or agave. Let it rest for 30 minutes.

3. After 30 minutes, taste again. Add lemon, honey, or mint as you see fit. If you add more mint, let it rest 30 more minutes, and try it again.

4. After you're satisfied with the taste, strain it and store it in a jar in the refrigerator.

Lemon Olive Oil Dressing

Beth
Yield: 1½ cups
Phase 1

Since Ivan chose to forgo vinegar on the menu during his healing phase, he has become very attached to this dressing. We use this blend on scrambled eggs, fish, grains, and, of course, salads. We even take it with us on the plane in 3-ounce jars when we travel.

Ingredients:

1 cup extra-virgin olive oil
⅓ cup lemon juice, freshly squeezed
1 small clove garlic, minced
½ teaspoon lemon zest, finely grated
½ teaspoon sea salt
¼ teaspoon cayenne
¼ teaspoon dry mustard

Instructions:

1. Whisk all ingredients together in a small bowl or spoon into a jar and shake to blend.

2. Taste and adjust salt and cayenne pepper to taste.

3. If the dressing is too zingy for you, feel free to add more olive oil to soften the flavor. A bit more salt will help temper the acid kick, too.

4. Use immediately or store, covered and chilled, up to 1 week (olive oil will solidify in the refrigerator, but it will melt quite quickly again at room temperature).

Shake well before serving.

Variation: make another Phase 1 version with grated fresh ginger, and add it to the lemon olive oil instead of the salt and garlic. The ginger version is especially good when served over bok choy, cabbage, or asparagus. Or if you are in a hurry, just mix the oil and lemon. It tastes great just like that.

Tip: experiment with mixing 1:1; you may like the lemon flavor more forward for your foods.

Special request: We beg you to please use only fresh lemon juice! The stuff you find in the little plastic lemons in the grocery store in no way resembles real lemon juice. Check the labels on those plastic lemons (and limes). You will find more in there than juice, in our experience.

Olive Oil Mayonnaise

Chef Eddie
Yield: 1¼ cups
Phase 3

In doing my research, I discovered a technique new to me on how to make mayonnaise using an immersion blender or, as we say in South Louisiana, a boat motor. Put the ingredients in a container just bigger than the head of the blender and deep enough to hold everything. Turn on the blender and boom! You have mayo. Fantastic.

Once you make fresh mayonnaise, you won't buy it from the store again. This mayonnaise is the base for many things and is on the Misner Plan. Use fresh farm eggs if you can get your hands on them. There is a noticeable difference.

Ingredients:
1 egg yolk
1 tablespoon lemon juice, freshly squeezed
1 tablespoon water
1 teaspoon mustard powder
1 cup olive oil, expeller pressed (extra-virgin will have a strong olive taste)
Kosher salt, to taste

Instructions:
1. Place the egg yolk, lemon juice, water, and mustard powder in a narrow, tall container. Pour the olive oil in and let it settle for a moment.

2. Using an immersion blender, process until the mayo starts to form. Once you start seeing mayo, gently move the blender up and down. Continue until all the oil is emulsified and the texture is thick.

3. Season to taste with kosher salt. You can store the mayo in the refrigerator up to several weeks.

Tip: To make variations on our basic mayonnaise, add fresh, chopped basil leaves or fresh, chopped cilantro, and even your favorite chili powder. Experiment with the combinations to discover what pleases your palate the most. You might also like to create dressings with the basic mayo by adding a bit of goat's milk, crushed garlic, and one of our spice mixes. This would make a great dip for veggies.

Pepper Greens Dressing

Chef Eddie
Yield: 1 cup
Phase 1

Fresh and packed full of nutrients, this dressing is excellent over fresh salad greens, crisp cucumbers, and even shrimp. Use watercress or arugula. Both will give you a peppery punch with a bitter green edge. This dressing really works well over a piece of fish or some shrimp, and it will add some variety to pour over your roasted or raw vegetables. On one of my trips to Rome, the bar snack in the hotel was little pieces of Parmigiano Reggiano with a bowl of arugula leaves next to it together with a jar of fantastic extra-virgin olive oil. The trick to the snack was to wrap the cheese with the arugula and dip in some oil. Seemed strange at first, but I know we didn't leave any. Simple and amazing, and fully approved for Phase 3!

Ingredients:
½ cup arugula leaves and stalks
½ cup lemon juice, freshly squeezed
2 teaspoons sea salt
¼ cup grapeseed oil

Instructions:
1. Combine all ingredients in a blender and process until you get the consistency you want. If it's too thick, and you don't want to load up on calories, add some Vegetable Stock instead of more oil.

2. Adjust the seasoning, and you are ready to go.

Tip: Watercress and arugula can be very peppery, which is what makes it so amazing. So be sure to taste it before you start adding any ground pepper to the salad on which you are pouring this delicious dressing.

Portuguese Hot Sauce

Chef Eddie
Yield: 2½ cups
Phase 3

This is a take on the traditional piri-piri sauce of the Portuguese. Hot and exotic, it's typically used on chicken, but be creative. It tastes really good with beans, on avocados and raw vegetables, or in guacamole. If you have this around, you never have to worry about dull food—that's for sure.

Ingredients:

2¼ cups extra-virgin olive oil
3 jalapeño peppers, coarsely chopped, stems, seeds, and all
2 poblano peppers, coarsely chopped, stems, seeds, and all
1 tablespoon crushed red pepper
1 teaspoon sea salt
1 tablespoon garlic, minced

Instructions:

1. Combine all ingredients except garlic in a saucepan over high heat. Cook, stirring, for 4 minutes. Stir in garlic, remove from heat, and allow it to cool to room temperature.

2. When the mixture is cool, pour it into a food processor bowl and pulse several times until smooth.

3. Strain the sauce through a fine-mesh strainer.

4. Pour the sauce into a glass container and cover it.

5. Let it sit for 1 week before using.

Tip: Keep your fire extinguisher handy. This one is *hot!*

Roasted Garlic

Chef Eddie
Yield: 1¼ cup
Phase 1

This is a 2-for-1 recipe. Roast the garlic in the oil, allow to cool, and you will have nicely roasted garlic and a portion of roasted garlic oil to use in your next mayo, salad dressing, or to cook your chicken. Not a bad deal, if you ask me.

Ingredients:

10-20 garlic cloves, peeled
Olive oil to cover to right below the tops of the cloves
Salt
Cayenne to taste
2 thyme or rosemary sprigs

Instructions:

1. Preheat oven to 300°F.

2. In a ramekin or other oven container just big enough to contain the cloves, pour olive oil over garlic cloves until covered about three-quarters of the way up.

3. Salt and pepper the cloves, add the herbs, and bake for 35 to 40 minutes or until cloves feel soft when pressed, and they are brown on the top.

4. Remove the garlic from the oil and set aside. Allow to cool, and then store in a jar for later use.

Roasted Shallots

Chef Eddie
Serves: 2
Phase 1

These are like candy. When you roast them, the natural sugars really come forward. Save the roasting oil to use in another dish. I like to mix these with sautéed mushrooms or mix them in with green beans. It will be all you can do to not eat them all before you are able to use them in your dish. All of a sudden, people will start appearing to "help" you out in the kitchen.

Ingredients:
2 large shallots, peeled
¼ cup grapeseed oil
¼ teaspoon kosher salt
⅛ teaspoon cayenne pepper

Instructions:
1. Preheat oven to 350°F.

2. In small, oven-safe bowl, coat both shallots with grapeseed oil and then pour remaining oil over them. (Oil should cover about ¼ of shallots.)

3. Sprinkle salt and cayenne pepper over each piece.

4. Cover them with foil. Place them in the oven for 45 minutes.

5. Take them out and remove foil. Put them back into oven for another 30 minutes. You will have two nicely browned shallots at this point.

6. Remove them from the oven and set aside to cool. Reserve the oil and toss shallots with it before serving.

Santa Fe Crema

Chef Eddie
Yield: ¾ cup
Phase 2

This is a lighter replacement for sour cream, so use it when you would normally use sour cream. You can change up the flavor by using Italian seasoning instead of Santa Fe Seasoning Mix.

Ingredients:
½ teaspoon lime juice
½ cup yogurt, goat's or sheep's milk
1 teaspoon Santa Fe Seasoning Mix, Phase 1 variation
¼ medium red onion, minced
⅓ cup cilantro, chopped
½ teaspoon sea salt

Instructions:
1. Mix all ingredients together in a bowl.

2. Let the mixture sit for a half hour, refrigerated. Adjust seasoning to taste.

Santa Fe Seasoning Mix

Chef Eddie
Yield: ¾ cup
Phase 3

Depending on where you live, this can be a very unique and flavorful spice blend to use. My first trip to Santa Fe, New Mexico, opened my eyes to a whole new world of exciting flavors and food preparations. At the base of many of those incredible flavors were the spices in this blend.

You'll be happy when you use this on chicken, certain fish, scallops, and even lobster.

Ingredients:
2 tablespoons chili powder, ancho or pure
2 teaspoons fresh ground cumin
2 tablespoons paprika (omit for Phase 1)
1 tablespoon fresh ground coriander seed
1½ teaspoons cayenne pepper
1 tablespoon garlic powder
1 teaspoon crushed red pepper
1 tablespoon sea salt
1 tablespoon dried oregano

Instructions:
1. Combine all ingredients in a bowl and whisk them together until well incorporated.

2. Store the mixture in an airtight container.

Sauce Piquant

Chef Eddie
Yield: 4 cups
Phase 3

In Louisiana this sauce is famous with rabbit, but you can use chicken or shrimp and love it just as much. You can also use it as a Diablo sauce.

Ingredients:
Extra-virgin olive oil
1 large onion, chopped
1 green bell pepper, chopped
1 jalapeño pepper, seeded and minced
1 tablespoon garlic, minced
2 tablespoons fresh thyme, chopped
2 tablespoons fresh oregano
2 cups tomatoes, peeled, seeded, and chopped
4 bay leaves
1 tablespoon Creole Seasoning Mix
Pinch crushed red pepper
3 cups Chicken Stock
Sea salt, to taste
Black pepper, freshly ground, to taste
3 tablespoons parsley, finely chopped

Instructions:
1. Heat olive oil in heavy-bottomed saucepan over high heat.

2. Add onions, green pepper, jalapeños, garlic, thyme, and oregano. Season with salt and pepper and sauté for 2 minutes.

3. Stir in tomatoes, bay leaves, Creole Seasoning Mix, a pinch of crushed red pepper, and Chicken Stock. Season with salt and pepper to taste, bring to a boil, and cook for 5 minutes.

4. Reduce heat and simmer for 20 minutes, then remove from heat. Pour mixture into a food processor and drizzle in olive oil while motor is running until it reaches the consistency of a rich tomato sauce. Pour mixture back in the saucepan and stir in parsley. Serve warm.

Thai Cashew Butter Sauce

Chef Eddie
Yield: ¼ cup
Phase 3

Think of this as a better replacement for that peanut sauce you're used to eating. You can make a satay dish with it or use it with vegetables as a dip. But the Thai Cashew Slaw and its variation, Thai Quinoa Pilaf, recipes are ones you will crave. This sauce is the base for those salads. I like to just have some sitting around like a jar of peanut butter that I can use on whatever I want.

Ingredients:
1 cup Homemade Nut Butter, cashew
4 tablespoons maguey sap or honey
2⅔ tablespoons ginger, freshly grated
¾ tablespoon Bragg's Liquid Aminos
2 teaspoons lime juice, freshly squeezed
½ teaspoon cayenne

Instructions:
1. Add Homemade Nut Butter, cashew and maguey sap or honey to a small saucepan and heat at low temperature to soften.

2. Add ginger, Bragg's Aminos, lime juice, and cayenne and stir until the mixture is smooth and creamy.

Tip: if you want a thinner dressing, simply stir in 1–2 teaspoons of water or olive oil.

Vegan Worcestershire Sauce

Chef Eddie
Yield: 3 cups
Phase 3

I have to admit, when I started looking for a Worcestershire sauce replacement, I would never have guessed a vegan one would work. In South Louisiana, Worcestershire sauce is a must, almost a mother sauce. Many famous dishes have it, or are based on it, including the renowned barbeque shrimp. It's so important that the good restaurants make it themselves and would never use that stuff in the bottle with the paper wrapper.

The difference is amazing. Store-bought Worcestershire sauce is a mixture of a lot of corn syrup, cane syrup, vinegar, cloves, peppers, anchovies, a little horseradish, and who knows what else, depending on who makes it. Obviously, that's no good for our plan.

I tried a few different ones while researching, but they left me a little underwhelmed. As it happened, I figured out the missing link. It had to do with reducing the vinegar. Once I figured that out, I had a killer sauce that I am really happy with.

A word of caution: reducing vinegar is a stinky process. My wife was not too happy with me, so if you can, do it outside! If you cannot, make sure your stove vent is on, and then diffuse some essential oil in your kitchen afterward.

Ingredients:
2 cups Bragg's apple cider vinegar
½ cup Bragg's Liquid Aminos
⅔ cup raw agave
1 teaspoon ground ginger
1 teaspoon ground yellow mustard seed (alternative, dry mustard)
1 teaspoon onion powder
1 clove garlic, crushed
½ teaspoon ground cinnamon
½ teaspoon cayenne pepper

Instructions:

1. Place apple cider vinegar in a saucepan over medium heat and reduce by half to about 1 cup.

2. Place the remaining ingredients in saucepan. Bring to a boil over medium-high heat. Reduce heat to simmer and cook until all liquid is reduced by half, about 20 minutes. This is the secret to success: reduce vinegar twice.

3. Strain the mixture through a fine-mesh sieve and let it cool completely before using.

Tip: this Vegan Worcestershire Sauce may be stored in an airtight container, refrigerated, for up to 3 months.

Twenty-Two

Phase 1 Food List

* Do not eat if there are active cancer cells in the body.
+ Especially good for people with active cancer cells.

VEGETABLES (ORGANIC) FOR DAYS 1–8

Prepare steam fried, steamed, or raw. Occasionally brushing veggies with grapeseed or tea seed oil and grilling on an infrared gas grill is OK. Do not allow them to burn:

Artichoke
Asparagus
Broccoli+ (including sprouts)
Brussels sprouts+
Cabbage+ (including bok choy+ and broccoli rabe+)
Cauliflower+
Celery, including celery root, or celeriac
Cilantro
Cucumber
Garlic+
Grape leaves

Green vegetables (leafy greens, green beans, zucchini, spinach, mustard greens, and collard greens)
Kale+, including sea kale
Kohlrabi
Kombu
Nori
Okra
Olive (in water with sea salt only, no brine, vinegar, or preservatives)
Onions+ (yellow, white, purple, all onion family vegetables, including scallions [a.k.a. green onions], shallots, and leeks)
Parsley, all types
Radish+
Rhubarb
Sprouts
Summer squash (yellow, Italian, Mexican gray)
Watercress+

No avocados
No beans
No beets
No carrots
No corn
No eggplant
No jicama
No mushrooms
No parsnips
No peas
No peppers
No potatoes
No rutabagas
No soybeans
No tomatoes
No yams
No winter squash, such as acorn, butternut, or spaghetti
No fermented vegetables, such as sauerkraut, kimchi, or miso

WHOLE COMPLEX GRAINS (ORGANIC) FOR DAYS 5–8

Cooked until chewy, not crunchy or soggy:

Amaranth

Brown rice

Buckwheat

Millet

Quinoa

Teff

Pilaf (with garlic, onions)

No white rice of any type, including risotto

No couscous or faro "rice"

No oats

No gluten grains (wheat, spelt, kamut, and barley)

No wild rice (which is a seed, not a grain)

SEASONINGS AND HERBS (ORGANIC) FOR DAYS 1–8

Cayenne and red pepper flakes

Cilantro, fresh or dry

Cinnamon

Dill

Garlic

Ginger (peeled and freshly grated)

Lemon juice, fresh squeezed

Mint

Oregano, fresh

Parsley, fresh

Rosemary, fresh

Sea salt

Stevia leaf, whole

No stevia extract

No sugars of any kind (including honey, syrup, molasses, sap, agave, raw, brown, sucrose, fructose, xylitol, beet, and coconut)

No vinegars or foods containing, or having been marinated in, vinegar

No soy sauce or tamari

LEGUMES/PULSES (ORGANIC): NONE DURING PHASE 1

FRUITS (ORGANIC) FOR DAYS 1–8
Lemon

OILS (ORGANIC) FOR DAYS 1–8
All oils, except those indicated, should be used cold, added to foods after cooking:
Citrus oils (used by the drop for flavoring)
Flaxseed oil
Safflower oil

These oils may be used cold *and* for cooking:
Coconut oil (cooking at lower temperatures)
Ghee (cooking and baking)
Grapeseed oil (cooking, baking, and roasting)
Olive oil, extra-virgin (when fresh, use for cooking, baking, and roasting)
Red palm fruit oil, extra-virgin, cold-pressed organic (cooking, baking, and roasting)
Tea seed oil (cooking, baking, and roasting)
No canola oil
No peanut oil
No lard
No butter

BEVERAGES FOR DAYS 1–8
Clean, purified water
Green tea (1 cup per day)
Herbal teas: mint, raspberry leaf, chamomile, and Pau D'Arco

ANIMAL PROTEIN
None during Phase 1

RAW, SPROUTED NUTS (ORGANIC)
None during Phase 1

SEEDS/NIBS (ORGANIC)
None during Phase 1

MILK ALTERNATIVES (ORGANIC)
None during Phase 1

Breakfast, Anyone?

It may seem odd to eat veggies for breakfast, since you are not used to doing so. Most people are used to eating mainly simple carbs for breakfast (think muffins, croissants, bagels, and the like), and sometimes they might include an egg or two for protein. You may also be used to always eating something sweet for breakfast (think pancakes with syrup, sweet cereals, and oatmeal with brown sugar and raisins). A big part of the Misner Plan is focused on changing habits and tastes, so breakfast can be a larger adjustment for most people than any other part of the Misner Plan.

SUGGESTED BREAKFASTS

Chopped cucumber salad with green onion tops, Lemon Olive Oil Dressing, and sea salt.

Steamed spinach with Lemon Olive Oil Dressing, sea salt, and roasted garlic or garlic powder.

Steam-fried green beans with Lemon Olive Oil Dressing, sea salt, and roasted garlic or garlic powder.

Steamed cauliflower with a Phase 1 Pantry Dressing.

Grilled zucchini/Italian or yellow squash: slice the squash lengthwise, brush with grapeseed oil or coconut oil, and grill on a countertop grill (like a George Foreman Grill) until lightly browned.

Add grilled onions and/or roasted garlic pieces to any of the dishes.

What's for Lunch?

Lunch can be easier to plan and prepare, as some of us already have a salad habit set for lunch. The difference here is going to be not adding croutons, hard-boiled eggs, or any meats. That doesn't mean your salad has to be boring. With the addition of tasty Phase 1 Misner Plan dressings, any old salad can go from plain to fabulous in just minutes.

SUGGESTED LUNCHES

Mixed salad greens and fresh herbs with Lemon Olive Oil Dressing or Pepper Dressing.

Grilled zucchini/Italian or yellow squash sprinkled with cayenne pepper flakes and served with a side of steamed red cabbage.

String beans drizzled with zucchini/Italian squash puree "sauce" (blend steamed zucchini/Italian squash with roasted garlic or powdered garlic and sea salt to taste) and garnish with chopped parsley.

Cauliflower "steaks" (cut the cauliflower into ¼-inch slices, toss in olive oil, then roast at 325°F until lightly browned, turning halfway through) with roasted garlic pieces and sea salt to taste.

It's Suppertime!

Supper is usually the heartiest meal of the day for most people. With the Misner Plan, we are turning that on its head. We teach that it is best to eat breakfast like a king, lunch like a prince, and supper like a pauper. That is: eat a hearty breakfast, a substantial lunch, and a very light supper. As you progress through Phase 1, you will find that your appetite will meet this routine. Often a single-food dish will be satisfying for supper.

SUGGESTED SUPPERS

Steamed broccoli with cayenne pepper flakes, drizzled with Lemon Olive Oil Dressing

Oven-roasted asparagus and rosemary with cauliflower puree (blend steamed cauliflower with white pepper, roasted garlic or garlic powder, and sea salt)

Wilted greens (mixed collard, mustard, and spinach) with Lemon Olive Oil Dressing, sea salt, and chopped dill

Bok choy, steam-fried and slightly caramelized in coconut oil, served with safflower oil, chopped ginger, and sea salt

Blended Broccoli Soup

Green Machine Veggie Soup

Phase 1 Supplement Schedule
Upon Waking
1 Premier Digest (follow with one capsule every waking hour)

With Meals
2 Premier Cleanse (increase each day by 1 until you are taking 4 capsules with each meal)
1 Premier Clay
1 Premier Probiotics

After Meals
1 AloeMannan-FX

To aid body detoxification during Phase 1
Alternate one Medi-Clay-FX with one Medi-Soak Cleanse or Medi-Body Bath for a total of two baths per day.

Twenty-Three

Baby Bok Choy

Beth
Serves: 2

There are so many great veggies to choose from during Phase 1. Bok choy was new to us when we started the Misner Plan, and I had never cooked it. We like the texture of bok choy as well as the exotic flavor. We add interest to our bok choy by drizzling it with our Lemon Olive Oil Dressing before eating it.

Ingredients:
4 heads of bok choy, with ends cut and leaves separated
Sea salt

Instructions:

1. Steam-fry bok choy in a large skillet or a wok.

2. Allow the water to cook off and bring the bok choy to a point of light caramelization, tossing it frequently with a fork so the leaves do not burn.

3. Remove it from the heat and sprinkle with salt to taste.

Tip: to deepen the Pacific Rim flavor of this dish, finely chop 1 teaspoon of peeled ginger and toss with the bok choy just before serving.

Basic "Pasta"

Chef Eddie
Serves: 4

When considering a substitute for regular pasta, zucchini or yellow squash will surprise and delight you with its versatility in this recipe.

Ingredients:

4 large zucchini or yellow squash, washed
1 tablespoon coconut oil
Sea salt

Instructions:

1. On a mandoline or with a food processor, julienne zucchini or squash and place it in a colander. You can also use the curly fry attachment for creating spirals for more interest.

2. Add a few dashes of sea salt to vegetables and toss to coat. Allow them to sit in the sink for about 20 minutes. This will help some of the excess water drain out from zucchini.

3. After the 20 minutes are up, place zucchini in some paper towels and squeeze gently to remove any remaining moisture. This will make it more pasta-like.

4. To eat plain, heat coconut oil in a skillet, toss the zucchini in oil for 2 minutes, remove, and add sea salt to taste. Serve with roasted garlic pieces and Pepper Greens Dressing.

Phase 3 Variation: serve with any of the pasta sauces, toss for 2–3 minutes in the hot pan. Serve immediately. You can serve with our Veggie Meatballs, as well.

Note: During Phases 1 and 2, it is best to eat your veggies with the peel. If you are intending to use the pasta in a Phase 3 hot dish, you may wish to peel the zucchini first. The green skin will add a flavor that may not match your sauce. If you are intending to use the pasta in a Phase 3 cold dish, peeling is optional, depending on the flavors of the mixed ingredients.

Blended Asparagus Soup

Chef Eddie
Serves: 4

This is a great soup on a winter's day, but it can also be served cold in the summer.

Ingredients:

1½ pounds chopped asparagus, tough ends removed
2 teaspoons grapeseed oil
1 large yellow onion, diced
1 clove garlic, minced
Leaves from 1 sprig thyme
3 cups Vegetable Stock
½ teaspoon sea salt, to taste
Pinch of cayenne pepper or Creole Seasoning Mix

Instructions:

1. In a cast-iron pot, sauté the chopped asparagus in grapeseed oil over medium heat until slightly caramelized.

2. Stir in onions and cook until translucent. Stir in the garlic and add the thyme leaves and Vegetable Stock, cover loosely, and simmer until the asparagus is soft, about 10–15 minutes.

3. Remove it from the heat and cool slightly.

4. Transfer the soup to a blender and puree until smooth.

5. Strain the soup through a fine-mesh strainer into a saucepan. Discard any solids.

6. Add salt and cayenne pepper and give the soup a quick stir. Serve.

Phase 3 Variation: add 1 tablespoon goat's or sheep's milk yogurt and stir in at the end to finish with sea salt and cayenne pepper.

Blended Broccoli Soup

Beth
Serves: 4

When Ivan and I repeat Phase 1, a substantial, blended soup is very satisfying and filling. This soup has no cream, but it does have a creamy texture and is packed with flavor, I promise.

Ingredients:

2 cups broccoli, chopped
½ medium yellow onion, chopped
¼ teaspoon sea salt
⅛ teaspoon garlic powder
1 tablespoon extra-virgin olive oil
1 tablespoon lemon juice, freshly squeezed
Pinch of cayenne pepper
Red pepper flakes

Instructions:

1. Steam the onion and broccoli until bright green and tender when pierced with a fork, reserve the cooking water, rinse in cold water.

2. Process the broccoli and onion with cooking water until smooth in the food processor (add more purified water to get desired consistency).

3. Add sea salt, garlic powder, olive oil, lemon juice, and cayenne pepper, and pulse until mixed.

4. Pour into soup bowls and sprinkle red pepper flakes sparingly on the top of each bowl to garnish.

Phase 2 Variation: this soup may be served with seasoned ground turkey.

Breakfast Frittata

Beth
Serves: 4

On the days when Ivan and I have to start our days very quickly, I chop up the vegetables in this dish the night before, put it all together in the morning, and then let it bake while we do our morning cardio exercise. The added bonus is that we can have it again the next day or even later on the same day, if our schedules are too packed to allow for a freshly cooked meal. We have enjoyed this dish well past Phase 1. It shows up on our menu every couple of weeks.

Ingredients:

2 tablespoons coconut oil
½ red onion, diced
1 zucchini, diced small
5 asparagus spears, chopped
1 teaspoon Phase 1 Misner Plan seasoning mix of your choice
½ teaspoon sea salt
Pinch of white pepper, ground
8 eggs (with 6 yolks removed)

Instructions:

1. Preheat oven to 350°**F**. Place a round stoneware baking dish with coconut oil in the oven as it preheats.

2. Combine chopped vegetables in a medium mixing bowl. Sprinkle seasoning mix, sea salt, and white pepper over vegetables, and stir to distribute spices evenly.

3. In a separate mixing bowl, beat the eggs until frothy. Pour into a bowl with vegetables and stir together with a wooden spoon.

4. Pour the egg mixture into the heated baking dish and return to oven. Bake for about 25 minutes, or until the desired color is reached and the frittata is firm in the middle.

5. Cut into fourths. Serve each piece on small plate with a garnish of your choice.

Phase 3 Variation: add 10 baby bella mushrooms, cleaned and sliced small to the vegetable mixture.

Brussels Sprouts and Crispy Shallots Salad

Chef Eddie
Yield: 2 cups

I don't like brussels sprouts. I never served them, nor had I ever had any use for them. But when I got involved with this book, I figured I had to use all the vegetables available to me to provide interest and variety to the menu, so what the heck, I'll try them out again. What I discovered is, boy, was I wrong. I just never worked with them long enough to figure them out.

What I had always seen was steamed brussels sprouts, but, frankly, what's the point? The other ways I saw were covered or sautéed in bacon fat and then tossed in some Gorgonzola or other bleu cheese. Better, but I can sure think of better ways to use bacon and bleu cheese than to cover up the flavor of brussels sprouts.

So I decided if I couldn't find a way to eat them raw, I wouldn't use them. After a little research, I settled on grating them. You get the intense flavor without the (in my opinion) too dense texture of whole sprouts. Add a little Lemon Olive Oil and some Crispy Shallots, and now we have something I look forward to eating.

Ingredients:

2 cups brussels sprouts, grated
1 tablespoon extra-virgin olive oil
¼ teaspoon fine sea salt
Lemon Olive Oil Dressing, to taste
⅔ cup Crispy Shallots

Instructions:

1. Use a food processor with grating blade for this one if you have it. Using a box grater for these little guys may leave you with some roughed up knuckles.

2. Grate all brussels sprouts and then pour them into a bowl. Reprocess any large chunks that are left.

3. Add 1 teaspoon of extra-virgin olive oil and toss (the little bit of olive oil will help seasonings stick to the greens), then season with salt to taste.

4. Dress with the Lemon Olive Oil Dressing and top with Crispy Shallots.

Variation: Ivan and Beth enjoy brussels sprouts roasted whole and salted.

Caramelized Onions

Chef Eddie
Serves: 4 cups

You will want to master this one. This basic technique adds so much flavor, but it's often not executed properly. There is no go-fast method, so take your time, enjoy the smells, and even have a good glass of your favorite, um, herbal tea while it's cooking.

Ingredients:

Several medium or large onions, yellow, white, or red
Grapeseed oil, as needed
Ghee (clarified butter), as needed
Sea salt, to taste

Instructions:

1. Prepare onions by cutting off ends and removing skin. Cut onions in half lengthwise and place them cut side down on a cutting board. Slice the onions to the desired thickness.

2. Coat the bottom of a wide, heavy-bottomed sauté pan with ½ grapeseed oil and ½ ghee mixture (about 1 teaspoon per onion). Heat the pan on medium-high until the oil is shimmering.

3. Add onion slices and stir to coat onions with oil. Spread onions out evenly over pan and let them cook, stirring occasionally, for 30 minutes or more, stirring every few minutes. As soon as onions start sticking to the pan, let them stick a little and brown, but then stir them before they burn. The trick is to leave them alone long enough to brown, but not so long that they burn. After the first 20–30 minutes, you may want to lower the stove temperature a little, and add water if you find that onions are burning. A metal spatula will help you scrape up browned bits from the bottom of the pan as caramelizing continues. As onions cook down, you may find you need to scrape the pan every minute, instead of every few minutes. Continue to cook and scrape until the onions are a rich brown color.

4. Store in refrigerator for several days in an airtight container.

Celery Root Chips

Chef Eddie
Serves: 8

Make a pile of these for your next party. They are flavorful and good for you at the same time. Can't beat that. You can use this same recipe for just about any type of root chip. The secret is to salt them first and leech the water out. That will give you the crunch you're looking for.

Ingredients:
1 celery root, peeled
Sea salt
Misner Plan Seasoning Mix of your choice

Instructions:
1. Preheat oven to 375°F.

2. Slice celery root with a mandoline about 1/16 inch thick. Place slices on a baking sheet. Lightly spray with coconut oil. Excessively salt slices and let them sit for about 15 minutes.

3. Remove slices to a bowl and rinse well. Dry them with a paper towel to squeeze as much moisture out as possible.

4. Place the cookie cooling rack on a baking sheet, place the chips on cookie-drying rack, and spray them with coconut oil. Flip and spray the other side.

5. Sprinkle with seasoning mix of your choice.

6. Place the entire rack with veggies in a preheated oven, and bake them until almost crispy. Approximately 13–15 minutes.

7. Take chips out of oven and let them sit about 15 minutes to finish crisping. Use one of the hummus recipes as your dip.

You can make this recipe using many different vegetables like celery, cauliflower, asparagus spears, and (when in Phase 3) beets, and eggplant. Just remember, the thinner you slice them, the crispier they will become, so keep an eye on your cooking times for different veggies and how thick you cut them.

Chili Mint Green Beans with Cucumbers

Chef Eddie

Serves: 4–6

This Phase 1 dish is one you will reach for even beyond the detox. The sweet of the mint contrasting with the heat of the cayenne paired with the crunch of the beans and cucumbers is something to look forward to—and this is just Phase 1.

Ingredients:

1 pound green beans, ends trimmed
2 garlic cloves, chopped
2 tablespoons lemon juice, fresh squeezed
⅓ cup fresh mint leaves
3 tablespoons extra-virgin olive oil
¼ teaspoon salt
¼ teaspoon red pepper flakes
¼ teaspoon powdered cayenne pepper
¼ teaspoon mustard powder
¼ large cucumber

Instructions:

1. Prepare a large bowl of ice water and set it aside.

2. Blanch green beans by steaming them, then immediately plunge them into ice water. Swish the beans around until they're completely cool. Spread on a flour sack towel on your counter and pat dry thoroughly. Put the green beans in a shallow dish.

3. In a blender, combine garlic and lemon juice. Add mint leaves, olive oil, salt, red pepper, cayenne powder, and mustard powder and combine until the mixture is very smooth. Pour into small mixing bowl.

4. Slice the cucumber paper thin, skin on.

5. Pour the dressing over the green beans, add the cucumber slices, and toss to coat the vegetables thoroughly with the dressing. Let the mixture rest at least 30 minutes at room temperature before serving, or refrigerate overnight, covered and chilled.

Note: when chilled and allowed to marinate overnight, the beans will lose some of their vibrant green color, and they will develop a more complex, intense flavor.

Tip: always leave the skin on the cucumber for texture.

Crispy Garlic Chips

Chef Eddie
Yield: ¼ cup

These garlic chips can add just that bit of crunch and intense flavor that make a good dish go to great. Do not take your eye off them—it happens fast!

Ingredients:

2 garlic bulbs, cloves separated, skin removed, ends trimmed
Olive or grapeseed oil, enough to cover the bottom of your skillet about ¼ inch
Sea salt, to taste

Instructions:

1. Using a sharp knife, slice garlic cloves into very thin slices, about ¼ inch thick.

2. Add oil to a small to medium-size sauté pan, over medium-high heat.

3. When oil is hot, place garlic slices into the pan, allowing them to crisp. You'll know you are there when the edges brown. Quickly remove the slices to a paper towel to drain and crisp up. Add salt.

Crispy Shallots

Chef Eddie
Yield: 4 servings

Use these to add intensity and crunch without having a whole plate of fried food. You can use these as a topping for soups or fish.

Ingredients:

1 cup shallots, peeled and finely sliced into matchstick thickness
3 tablespoons grapeseed or coconut oil
Sea salt, to taste

Instructions:

1. Preheat heavy-bottomed, deep skillet to a medium-high heat, add about a ½ inch of oil to the pan, and bring to temperature.

2. Pull layers of the shallots apart. Place them by slotted spoon in heated oil for approximately 2–3 minutes. Look for a golden brown color.

3. Pour them out on a paper towel and spread them into a single layer.

4. Immediately sprinkle a little fine sea salt on all pieces and let them continue to crisp. Crisping time will depend on the humidity in your area.

Phase 2 Variation: you can use the Eddie's Caesar Dressing or any of the Misner Plan Olive Oil Mayonnaise variations as a dip or dressing.

Phase 3 Variation: add 1 tablespoon Pecorino Romano or Parmesan Cheese.

Tip: this is a great garnish to use when you are craving something else on your dish, such as bacon bits.

Green Machine Veggie Soup

Beth

Serves: 4

This soup has both blended and chunky features, making it perfect for Phase 1. It's filling and delicious.

Ingredients:

8 brussels sprouts
½ head of broccoli, including stalk
8 spears of asparagus, ends trimmed
1 small zucchini
¼ head of green cabbage, roughed chopped
¼ yellow onion, chopped
3 cloves garlic, mashed by the flat side of a knife until made into a paste
Sea salt
⅛ teaspoon garlic powder
⅛ teaspoon celery seed
Cayenne pepper, to taste

Instructions:

1. Steam until slightly tender: brussels sprouts and broccoli, including the stalk, chopped into smaller pieces; asparagus and zucchini chopped into five or six pieces.

2. In a blender or food processor, blend steamed vegetables with their cooking water until completely liquefied (keep the center hole on the blender lid open so lid does not pop off from the heat).

3. In a separate pan, steam until slightly tender: green cabbage, yellow onion, and garlic (reserve cooking water).

4. Add the blended veggies to the steamed veggies and add some cooking water to get the desired consistency.

5. Add to taste: sea salt, garlic powder, celery seed, and cayenne pepper.

6. After simmering for about 5 minutes, take the soup off the burner and serve immediately.

Tip: add about ⅛ cup of Lemon Olive Oil Dressing to your pot before serving.

Phase 2 Variation: add steam-fried ground turkey seasoned with organic Italian seasoning.

Phase 3 Variation: include chopped tomatoes with cabbage/onion mixture.

Grits

Chef Eddie
Serves: 4

Well, almost grits. For Phase 1, this is a great way to start the day or simply have a great between meal snack. You can have the cauliflower ready ahead of time to just put in the pan and quickly sauté.

Ingredients:
1 head cauliflower, stem and all
1 medium onion, minced
2 stalks celery, minced
1 tablespoon garlic, minced
Coconut or grapeseed oil
Ghee

Instructions:
1. Preheat oven to 375°F.

2. Roast cauliflower until nearly done. It should still have a little crunch to it and be just slightly brown on the outside. In a convection oven, this should take 15–20 minutes.

3. Remove cauliflower from oven, give it a rough chop, and place it in a food processor. Puree cauliflower to about the consistency and size of risotto. It is best to pulse the blade to get to this texture.

4. Preheat a cast-iron skillet with a little oil until you can see the heat rising from the pan.

5. Add onion and celery and cook for 2 minutes. Add garlic and 2 cups of cauliflower puree. Add sea salt and cayenne pepper to the mixture, 2 tablespoons ghee, and sauté until heated through. If it's a little too dry in the pan, you can add a touch of broth, olive oil, or some more ghee. The grits should brown up nicely.

6. Spoon the grits onto a plate. Serve immediately.

Tip: for a twist, add a little fresh spinach toward the end of cooking.

Phase 2 Variation: add a poached egg to get the creaminess of the yolk mixed in with the buttery cauliflower. Add a little garnish of goat cheese, and you have a great breakfast.

Indonesian Cauliflower

Chef Eddie
Serves: 4

The horseradish added to the cauliflower is what makes this dish head and shoulders above just your plain, ordinary cauliflower plate. One of the keys to success in Phase 1 is to make your meals vibrant and hearty with big, bold flavors. Detoxing doesn't have to be boring!

Ingredients:

3 tablespoons coconut oil, melted
4 tablespoons Indonesian Spice, toasted
1 cauliflower head, chopped
6 cloves roasted garlic
½ teaspoon lemon zest

Instructions:

1. Preheat oven to 375°F.

2. Line a baking sheet with parchment paper.

3. In a large bowl, mix melted coconut oil and toasted spices.

4. Add cauliflower, garlic cloves, and lemon zest. Stir until all florets are well coated with oil.

5. Spread the cauliflower mixture onto prepared baking sheet and bake for 25 minutes.

Phase 3 Variation: serve with fresh Horseradish Dill Dip.

Kale Chips

Chef Eddie
Yield: 2½ cups

When you need something crunchy and satisfying for a snack, these kale chips fit the bill. Be sure to lightly coat each leaf of kale with oil. If you can mist them with an olive oil sprayer, all the better.

Ingredients:

1 small bunch kale, washed and dried completely and chopped into 2-inch pieces
2 tablespoons extra-virgin olive oil
Sea salt for sprinkling

Instructions:

1. Preheat oven to 275°F.

2. Remove the ribs from the kale and cut into pieces. Place the kale on a baking sheet and toss it with the olive oil, making sure to cover all parts of the kale with a little oil. As an alternative, you can spray it or rub each leaf individually (not recommended for your sanity, but it works) and salt. Bake until crisp, turning the leaves halfway through, about 20 minutes.

3. Feel free to season this with your favorite Phase 1 Misner Plan seasonings.

Phase 3 Variation: Creole Seasoning Mix and Santa Fe Seasoning Mix go well with these, but experiment with other spice blends.

Lemon and Artichoke "Pasta"

Chef Eddie
Serves: 2

The lemons and artichokes are delicious together and add variety to a basic dish, making it something to look forward to.

Ingredients:

1 cup zucchini squash ribbons (see below)
1 cup yellow squash ribbons
Grapeseed or tea seed oil
3 tablespoons yellow onion, minced
1 clove garlic, diced
⅓ cup artichoke hearts, diced (using frozen is OK)
⅛ teaspoon sea salt
¼ teaspoon crushed red pepper
⅓ cup fresh parsley, chopped
1½ teaspoons lemon juice
¼ cup fresh basil, chopped

Instructions:

1. Using a mandoline or food processor attachment, julienne the squash into linguine-size ribbons.

2. When you're finished julienning, sprinkle salt over the ribbons and place them in a colander in the sink for about 20 minutes. You want to get rid of excess water; otherwise, when you sauté the ribbons, you'll have a pan full of a watery mess. Squeeze them dry with paper towels.

3. Using a medium-size skillet, add enough grapeseed or tea seed oil to coat the bottom. Turn the burner to medium high and heat the pan until the oil is shiny and shimmers.

4. Add onion and sauté until it starts to brown slightly.

5. Add garlic and sauté for an additional 30 seconds.

6. Add squash ribbons, artichokes, salt, crushed red pepper, parsley, lemon juice, and basil, and toss until heated through. Remove from heat. Serve immediately.

Tip: if you're in a hurry and need a quick sauté, consider using Lemon Olive Oil Dressing as a substitute for the garlic, lemon juice, and herbs.

Lemon-Garlic Green Beans

Chef Eddie
Serves: 4

This recipe will keep green beans from ever being boring again. It turns a basic green veggie into something exciting, ensuring that the side dish will be as exciting as the entree. The lemon lends that bit of pop that makes it exciting.

Ingredients:
1 pound haricots verts (green beans), ends trimmed
1 tablespoon grapeseed oil
3 tablespoons ghee
2 garlic gloves, minced
1 teaspoon red pepper flakes
1 tablespoon lemon zest
1¼ tablespoons lemon juice, freshly squeezed
⅛ teaspoon sea salt
⅛ teaspoon cayenne pepper

Instructions:
1. Blanch green beans in large stockpot of well-salted, boiling water until bright green in color and tender crisp, roughly 2 minutes.

2. Drain and shock in a bowl of ice water to stop beans from cooking and preserve bright green color.

3. Place a large, heavy skillet over medium heat. Add oil and ghee and bring to temperature. Add garlic and red pepper flakes and sauté until fragrant, about 30 seconds.

4. Add green beans and continue to sauté until coated in ghee and heated through, about 5 minutes. Remove from heat.

5. Transfer to a serving bowl. Add lemon zest and lemon juice, season with salt and cayenne pepper, and toss to combine. Enjoy.

Middle Eastern Spinach Soup

Chef Eddie
Serves: 6

By simply adding some exotic spices to this dish, you are easily transported to a whole new stratosphere.

Ingredients:

1 tablespoon extra-virgin olive oil
1 medium onion, chopped
⅓ cup celery, finely diced
Sea salt, to taste
2 garlic cloves, minced
6 cups Vegetable Stock
A bouquet garni made with a bay leaf and a couple of sprigs each of thyme and parsley
1½ pounds fresh spinach, stemmed and washed thoroughly
¼ teaspoon ground allspice
⅛ teaspoon ground clove
⅛ teaspoon nutmeg, freshly grated
¼ teaspoon ground cinnamon
1 scant teaspoon coriander seeds, lightly toasted

Instructions:

1. Heat olive oil over medium heat in large, heavy soup pot or Dutch oven and add onion and celery. Cook, stirring until tender, about 5 minutes. Add a generous pinch of salt and garlic and cook until the garlic smells fragrant, 30 seconds to 1 minute.

2. Add stock and bouquet garni and bring to a boil. Reduce heat, cover, and simmer 30 minutes. Remove the thyme sprig and bay leaf. Stir in spinach and spices, cover, and simmer 5 minutes, stirring once or twice. The spinach should maintain its bright-green color.

3. Using an immersion blender, or a regular blender with the vent open, puree soup. Remember, hot soup will forcefully push the top off in a messy explosion if the blender is closed airtight, so leave center cap off. Return to the pot and heat through, stirring.

Phase 2 Variation: Use Chicken Stock instead of water after completing Phase 1. Whisk 1 cup of Greek goat's or sheep's milk yogurt into soup. Season to taste with sea salt. If you feel it needs a second cup of yogurt, add it, and then adjust the salt, if necessary.

Olive Tapenade

Chef Eddie
Yield: 1 cup

This classic tapenade recipe's secret is the quality of the olives you choose in the beginning. Keep handy for those times when you want to dress up your Phase 1 meals for more flavor. You will also really enjoy our tapenade during Phase 3 as a spread on any of our Misner Plan crackers or flat breads. Remember to buy olives packed in water in glass jars, not cans, please.

Ingredients:
1 cup black or green olives, pitted
4 garlic cloves, peeled
1 cup parsley, fresh
1 lemon, freshly juiced
⅛ teaspoon cayenne pepper
2 tablespoons extra-virgin olive oil
Sea salt, to taste

Instructions:
1. Place all ingredients together in a Vitamix or blender.

2. Blend until smooth.

Tip: keep this tasty tapenade in an airtight container in your fridge.

Ratatouille
(Well, Almost)

Chef Eddie
Serves: 4

This dish is not quite a jambalaya since there is no rice. And, yes, I know ratatouille has to-mato and this doesn't, but when you get to Phase 3, throw some in if they're in season, all right? Regardless of what you call it, this salad makes a great lunch, side dish, or light din-ner. Toss it with one of the dressings mentioned in the pantry section, and you can serve it warm or cold. Even better, you can pack yourself a container, bring your dressing with you in another, and have a meal at your office or on the go.

Ingredients:
Grapeseed oil, for cooking
1 large Spanish onion, sliced thinly
2 cloves garlic, chopped
1 small zucchini, roughly chopped
1 small yellow squash, roughly chopped
1 pound fresh asparagus spears, roughly chopped
4 to 6 artichoke hearts, quartered, rinsed of any residuals, and drained (optional, but really good)
⅛ cup extra-virgin olive oil
1 lemon, freshly juiced
½ cup fresh parsley, chopped
Sea salt, to taste
Cayenne pepper to taste

Instructions:
1. Drizzle 1 to 2 tablespoons of grapeseed oil into a medium-size sauté pan and place over medium-high heat. Add onion and sauté 1 to 2 minutes, stirring often. Add garlic to the pan and continue to cook 1 more minute.

2. Lower heat to medium low and add zucchini, yellow squash, asparagus, and artichoke hearts. Toss to coat vegetables evenly with onions and garlic. Cover, and let heat through 2 to 4 minutes.

3. Remove from heat and finish with the Misner Plan dressing of your choice or just use olive oil and fresh lemon juice to brighten it up.

Tip: Chop up some of your favorite herbs, such as parsley, cilantro, or mint, and use at the end. You can even fold in some cooked quinoa. Remember to pay attention to what phase you're in because there are many variations you can use here.

Roasted Cauliflower with Turmeric and Cumin

Beth Misner
Serves: 4

This warming and tasty delight makes a great breakfast that is both filling and delicious in Phase 1. The ingredients also can help the body reduce inflammation. Turmeric has very strong anti-inflammatory properties. When you add the flavor of cumin to that of the turmeric, your taste buds will be singing!

Ingredients:
1 head cauliflower
½ cup extra-virgin olive oil
1-inch piece of turmeric root
1-inch piece of ginger root
1 clove garlic
⅓ lemon
½ teaspoon ground cumin
¼ teaspoon sea salt
Cayenne pepper, to taste

Instructions:
1. Preheat oven to 350°F.

2. Prepare vegetables: wash cauliflower, cut into florets, and set aside. Wash turmeric and ginger roots (do not peel), cut into small chunks; peel garlic clove; cut end off lemon and discard, then slice remaining lemon into three pieces.

3. Pour olive oil into small Bullet blender mixing cup. Add turmeric root, ginger root, garlic clove, lemon slices, cumin, and sea salt. Process until smooth.

4. Place cauliflower florets into large ziplock bag and pour turmeric sauce over them. Seal bag and toss so each piece is covered. Pour sauced cauliflower into a baking dish to make a

nice layer. Roast for 30 minutes. Check for tenderness and some browning. Return to oven, if needed, for 5-10 more minutes until dish reaches desired tenderness.

5. Serve plated with a dash of cayenne pepper, also known for its anti-inflammatory properties.

Phase 2 Variation: top this dish with poached eggs.

Phase 3 Variation: Roast cauliflower with 8-10 cherry tomatoes for a pop of color and added flavor. Add freshly ground black pepper to the sauce.

Tip: try the turmeric-cumin sauce with roasted zucchini, yellow squash, and even onions.

Southern Greens

Chef Eddie
Serves: 4 to 6

I grew up in the sixties in New Orleans way before the advent of grocery stores with wide vegetable offerings. In fact, I didn't even know there was another kind of lettuce other than iceberg until I was a late teenager in high school working at my friend's seafood restaurant. I would go with his dad, Drago Cvitanovich, to pick up oysters down the bayou in a town called Port Sulphur where the oyster boats docked. Like my friend's dad, all the fishermen were Croatian, and many of them had farms that grew all kinds of citrus and greens. Because of the common national tie, we would come back with the best sacks of oysters and big boxes of mustard, turnip, collards, and who-knows-what-other kind of greens that they would give him. Klara, my friend's mother, would cook them up in the restaurant, and we would eat greens all evening and into the rest of the week. To this day, as we say here in the South, I love me some greens!

Ingredients:

5 bunches of any greens like collard, mustard, chard, turnips
3 tablespoons olive or grapeseed oil
3 garlic cloves, sliced thin
1 large yellow onion, sliced
1–2 cups veggie broth
Sea salt, to taste
Cayenne pepper, powdered

Instructions:

1. Heat a cast iron Dutch oven over medium-high heat. When hot, add oil and sliced onion; season with salt and cook for 5 minutes or until onions are soft.

2. Add garlic and cayenne pepper and cook for another minute. Add greens, in batches if necessary, with about ¼ cup of veggie broth with each batch. Cook them, stirring frequently, until they begin to wilt. Bring to a simmer; cook greens for 12 to 14 minutes or until they are tender and most of the liquid has evaporated.

Tips: Later on when you can have it, add a bit of apple cider vinegar at the end. Be sure to use just enough salt and pepper to enhance the greens and let their natural flavors shine. Also, go moderate on the broth, using just enough to braise the greens. They will release liquid on their own. If you overdo it a bit, and the greens are too mushy, add more broth and make soup!

Steamed Lemon Spinach

Beth
Serves: 2

Spinach always seemed so boring before we created the Misner Plan. Adding flavors and seasonings to such a healthy veggie makes us crave spinach now.

Ingredients:
Purified water
1 pound fresh baby spinach
1 tablespoon Lemon Olive Oil Dressing
Sea salt flakes, to taste
Garlic powder, to taste

Instructions:
1. In a large skillet or wok, bring ½ inch of purified water to a gentle boil.

2. Add fresh spinach leaves and allow them to lightly steam just until wilted.

3. Drain and toss with Lemon Olive Oil Dressing. Add sea salt flakes and garlic powder to taste.

Vegetable Stock

Chef Eddie
Yield: 2 quarts

Whenever possible, you want to cook with a good stock. Using this stock will add depth when you cook rice in a rice cooker. Good stock is often the element that makes a huge difference between a mediocre dish and a really great dish. You can even poach fish in it.

Ingredients:
1 tablespoon grapeseed oil
2 large onions
4 stalks celery, including some leaves
2 bunches scallions, chopped
8 cloves garlic, minced
20 sprigs fresh parsley
12 sprigs fresh thyme
4 bay leaves
2 teaspoons sea salt
4 quarts water

Instructions:
1. Chop scrubbed vegetables into 1-inch chunks. Remember, the greater the surface area, the more quickly vegetables will yield their flavor.

2. Heat oil in a soup pot. Add onion, celery, scallions, garlic, parsley, thyme, and bay leaves. Cook over medium-high heat for 5–10 minutes, stirring frequently.

3. Add salt and water and bring to a boil. Lower heat and simmer uncovered for 30 minutes. Strain. Reserve vegetables to serve later.

Veggie Bowl

Chef Eddie
Yield: 1½ cups

This is meant to be a quick, easy dish for a great lunch without a whole lot of effort. You can even add some Veggie Stock and blend this one quickly into a soup.

Ingredients:
2 tablespoons grapeseed oil
⅓ cup brussels sprouts, chopped
⅓ cup celeriac, peeled and chopped
⅓ cup red onion, chopped
⅓ cup broccoli, chopped (include some stem pieces)
⅓ cup zucchini, chopped
1 sprig thyme, fresh
Sea salt, to taste
1 teaspoon Creole Seasoning Mix

Instructions:
1. Preheat grapeseed oil in a pan over medium heat. Add brussels sprouts and cook for about 3–4 minutes. Add celeriac to the pan and cook for about 3 minutes, stirring often. Cooking time will depend on the size of the chopping you did. Taste a brussels sprout and a celeriac piece to see if they are done.

2. Add red onions, broccoli, and zucchini. Sprinkle fresh thyme, coarse sea salt, and the Creole Seasoning Mix over the cooking veggies and mix well.

3. Cook for another 5 minutes, or until the veggies are browned and softened. Remove from heat and enjoy.

Tip: try variations on the spice mixtures—Indonesian Seasoning Mix or Santa Fe Seasoning Mixes.

Zucchini Chips

Chef Eddie
Yield: 3 cups

This dish will satisfy your salt and crunch cravings, and you won't feel like you missed anything at all.

Ingredients:
5 medium zucchini, cut into ⅛-inch slices
2 tablespoons sea salt
3 tablespoons grapeseed oil
2½ tablespoons dried basil
3 tablespoons dried rosemary
1½ tablespoons dried marjoram
½ teaspoon thyme

Instructions:
1. Preheat oven to 325°F.

2. Sprinkle sliced zucchini with salt and place in a colander in the sink for about 15–20 minutes. This will begin to sweat the water from the vegetables and help the chips to crisp. Remove from colander and press with paper towels to dry off the moisture.

3. In a large bowl, combine grapeseed oil and spices and mix well.

4. Place zucchini slices in the bowl and toss to completely coat with oil and spice mixture.

5. Place chips on a cooling rack, transfer into oven, and bake slices for 30 minutes. Check for browning. When slices are lightly browned, remove one from the oven and set aside until you can taste it. If it is semicrisp, they are ready. Remove the slices from oven and let them cool down. They will crisp up further as they cool.

Tip: Try a small batch first. Oven temperatures vary, all zucchini are different, and convection ovens reduce the time and add crispness. Try a small batch in your oven and see what the timing is for you

Twenty-Four

Artichoke Fennel Quinoa

Chef Eddie
Yield: 1¼ cups

Although in the later phases you could use this as a side dish, it is very satisfying and will completely satiate your hunger in Phase 1. The flavors are interesting and lend themselves well to be influenced in a wide variety of ways.

Ingredients:
1 cup sprouted quinoa, cooked and lightly salted
¼ cup artichoke hearts, cooked and diced
2 teaspoons Lemon Olive Oil Dressing
2 tablespoons fennel, diced
4 tablespoons fresh parsley, roughly chopped
Sea salt, to taste
¼ teaspoon cayenne
¼ cup mint
1 teaspoon lemon juice, freshly squeezed

Instructions:

1. Combine all ingredients in a mixing bowl and toss together.

2. Adjust seasoning to taste. It should taste bright and fresh. If it's a little flat, spritz with some more lemon juice.

Cinnamon Quinoa

Chef Eddie
Serves: 2

In an attempt to make something a little more breakfastlike, I came up with this dish. I think it will work equally well with millet and may even lend itself to be a little creamier, particularly when you can add a little coconut milk to it. As it sits, though, it's Phase 1 friendly.

Ingredients:

1 cup sprouted quinoa, prepared and lightly salted
2 tablespoons coconut oil, melted
½ teaspoon cinnamon
¼ teaspoon nutmeg

Instructions:

1. Combine all ingredients and toss in a bowl until quinoa is coated well with coconut oil and spices.

2. Adjust salt to taste and serve.

Tip: scrape the inside of a vanilla bean and stir in for more variety.

Phase 3 Variation: serve with coconut or hazelnut milk.

Quinoa Florentine

Beth
Serves: 2

Varying the types of grains we eat during Phase 1 is important. Ivan discovered he really likes quinoa, an ancient grain that has gained a new following.

Ingredients:

1 cup sprouted quinoa
⅓ yellow onion, diced
1 tablespoon coconut oil
1 clove garlic, minced
½ teaspoon Italian seasoning
1 cup fresh baby spinach leaves
Sea salt flakes, to taste

Instructions:

1. Simmer quinoa in water over until grains begin to pop open.

2. While quinoa cooks, sauté onions in coconut oil until transparent. Just before removing from heat, add garlic and Italian seasoning and stir together until veggies begin to caramelize ever so slightly.

3. Before water cooks completely off quinoa, add baby spinach leaves and gently fold in until wilted. Remove from heat.

4. Stir in sautéed onions and garlic.

5. Spoon into bowls and finish with sea salt flakes to taste.

Phase 3 Variation: use wild rice instead of quinoa and add some chopped tomatoes and ground turkey, too.

Steam-Fried Veggie Breakfast Bowl

Beth
Serves: 2

Eating grains during the second half of Phase 1 makes breakfast more interesting. Even after Phase 1, we make it a point to eat grains for breakfast from time to time. This recipe is good with a variety of vegetables. Watch for what is in season at your farmers' market and experiment with asparagus, scallions, broccolini, and cauliflower. The onions and garlic are good to include year-round for their strong, cancer-fighting compounds.

Ingredients:
1 cup sprouted nongluten grains of choice
½ cup broccolini, chopped
½ cup zucchini, chopped
¼ yellow onion, diced
1 clove of garlic, minced
Sea salt, to taste

Instructions:
1. Steam grains in 1 cup of purified water for 8–10 minutes or until al dente.

2. Steam-fry vegetables until tender.

3. Combine grains with veggies and add sea salt to taste. For extra depth, add some Lemon Olive Oil Dressing.

Phase 3 Variation: add tomatoes and let them simmer with veggies.

Tabbouleh

Chef Eddie
Serves: 4

I looked high and low to try to find some inspiration to elevate the basic tabbouleh recipe, but I guess when it's just right, you don't mess with it. What you see here is pretty much the standard recipe with sprouted quinoa substituted for the bulgur wheat, and no tomato for a Phase 1 dish.

Ingredients:
2 cups sprouted quinoa, prepared
⅓ cup lemon juice, freshly squeezed
⅓ cup extra-virgin olive oil
4 garlic cloves, minced
1 teaspoon sea salt
1 medium cucumber, peeled and cut into cubes
1 red onion, diced fine
½ cup parsley, finely chopped
1 cup spinach, chopped
1 cup fresh mint, finely chopped
1 cup watercress, roughly chopped

Instructions:
1. In small bowl, whisk together lemon juice, oil, garlic, and salt, and pour over prepared quinoa.

2. Add the remaining ingredients and toss well.

3. Cover and refrigerate for at least 30 minutes before serving.

Tropical Brown Rice

Chef Eddie
Serves: 2

Using fresh herbs and high-quality coconut oil will make this recipe one of your favorites. Get used to having fresh herbs around all the time.

Ingredients:

1½ tablespoons coconut oil, melted
2 cups sprouted brown rice, precooked, seasoned with sea salt
2 tablespoons mint, roughly chopped
2 tablespoons cucumber, finely diced

Instructions:

1. Add coconut oil to small skillet and heat to medium-high heat; stir in brown rice until well coated with oil.

2. Add mint (reserve some for garnishing) and let it cook for 1 minute.

3. Plate and garnish with diced cucumber and mint.

Twenty-Five

Foods to Add in Phase 2 (All Phase 1 Foods Are Used as Well)

ANIMAL PROTEIN

Cheese, goat's or sheep's milk only with no mold inhibitors, such as natamycin, and only if you have no inflammatory conditions

Eggs, organic, pasture raised when possible (1 yolk per 3 whites)

Poultry, antibiotic- and hormone-free, about once every 2 weeks

Chicken
Turkey

Seafood, should be wild caught and not farmed

Cod
Flounder
Haddock
Lobster
Salmon
Scallops

Shrimp
White fish

Yogurt, plain, organic (goat's or sheep's milk when possible, and only if you have no inflammatory conditions)

Phase 2 Supplement Schedule

WITH MEALS
2 Premier Digest
1 Premier Clay
1 Premier Probiotics

To maintain body detoxification during Phase 2, enjoy one Medi-Clay-FX and one Medi-Body Bath each week. It is suggested you space your baths evenly; for example: Sunday, Medi-Clay-FX, and Thursday, Medi-Body Bath.

Twenty-Six

Bammilicious Buckwheat Pancakes

Beth
Yield: 10 4-inch pancakes

The delicious addition of buckwheat to the gluten-free-flour mix creates a pancake you will be tempted to eat frequently, but remember, you are still resetting your body in Phase 2, so resist the urge to make a double batch. This is a great Sunday morning brunch recipe that the whole family will enjoy.

Ingredients:
1 cup gluten-free flour blend
½ cup buckwheat flour
½ cup brown rice flour
2 teaspoons Homemade Baking Powder
1 teaspoon baking soda
¼ teaspoon sea salt
3 egg whites
1 cup plain yogurt, goat's or sheep's milk

Grapeseed oil, for cooking
Coconut oil, to taste

Instructions:

1. Take eggs and yogurt out of the refrigerator before beginning. Break the eggs into a bowl, cover, and allow them to come to room temperature. Separate the eggs but do not reserve the yolks unless you are close to the end of Phase 2 and want to use them to make mayonnaise.

2. Stir together the dry ingredients in a medium-size mixing bowl.

3. Whisk together the wet ingredients in a small mixing bowl.

4. Add the wet ingredients to the dry ingredients and mix quickly and thoroughly.

5. Heat a cast iron skillet over medium-high heat and add a spoonful of grapeseed oil.

6. Ladle the batter ¼ cup at a time into skillet and cook until browned lightly on both sides.

7. While still warm, spread the pancakes with coconut oil after cooking, and serve immediately.

Phase 3 Variation: include ⅛ cup of your favorite natural sweetener (applesauce, honey, raw agave, coconut nectar, or maguey sap) with the wet ingredients and add 1 mashed banana and ¼ cup of chopped pecans to the batter before cooking. Serve topped with pureed stone fruit (apricots, peaches, and plums) or yogurt with cinnamon.

Cauliflower Tortillas

Chef Eddie
Yield: 6

These creative tortillas make a good base for a lot of things, from fish tacos to a veggie wrap.

Ingredients:

1 head cauliflower
2 eggs
Sea salt, to taste
Cayenne pepper, to taste
2 teaspoons Santa Fe Seasoning Mix
Ghee for cooking

Instructions:

1. Preheat oven to 375°F and line a baking tray with parchment paper.

2. Cut up a head of cauliflower (with most of the stem removed) into pieces that will fit into a food processor. Blanch them by placing them into a pot of rapidly boiling water for 2–3 minutes. Drain water and remove cauliflower to a bowl of ice water to let it cool for about 2–3 minutes. Drain and dry thoroughly.

3. In small batches, pulse the cauliflower in the food processor until you get a texture slightly finer than rice. You should end up with about 2 packed cups.

4. Place macerated cauliflower in a medium-size bowl and add two well-beaten eggs, Santa Fe Seasoning Mix, and a dash of salt and cayenne pepper. Mix until all ingredients are well combined. Batter may be a little bit runny, but shouldn't be pure liquid.

5. Spread mixture onto a baking sheet into 6 small fairly flat circles. Remember we are going for a tortilla-like shape and thickness, although these may be a touch thicker. Keep them fairly small, so they are easy to flip. The larger they get, the harder they are to flip.

6. Place in the oven for 10 minutes. Remove from the oven and carefully peel off the parchment. Flip them and place back in the oven for 5–7 more minutes.

7. When done, place on a wire rack to cool. Some people I have talked to like them just like this and don't get to the next step. After the tortillas have cooled, you can refrigerate them separated by pieces of parchment and use later.

8. Heat a medium-size pan over medium heat with a spoonful of ghee. When the ghee is hot and the pan is making some bubbles or a little noise, place the tortillas into the pan, pressing down slightly, and brown them to your liking, about 30 seconds per side. This extra step adds a lot to the presentation and gives it that buttery edge that is so good in fresh tortillas.

Tip: For a breakfast experience, substitute ground cinnamon and nutmeg for the cayenne pepper and Santa Fe Seasoning Mix. You may wish to cook them in red palm oil, instead of ghee, for another layer of flavor.

Chicken Bone Broth

Beth
Yield: 1 quart

There is nothing more healing, in my opinion, than a good bone broth. Allowing the chicken bones to simmer for so long extracts all the minerals and other healing properties from them. You will love the depth of flavor this broth lends to cooked grains, soups, and other dishes where Chicken Bone Broth is used. It is thicker than stock, so be aware of that if you use it in place of the stock. This bone broth is quite beneficial to feed to older dogs, too, since it is so full of glucosamine and chondroitin that it becomes gelatinous when cooled.

Ingredients:

1 chicken carcass with skin, meat removed
Water to cover

Instructions:
1. Place chicken bones and skin in large stockpot. Cover about 1 inch with purified water.

2. Heat water to a gently rolling boil. Cover stockpot and reduce heat so water will gently simmer.

3. Allow it to gently simmer for a minimum of 12 hours. If you are able, allow it to simmer for up to 30 hours. Be very sure the simmer is so gentle that the water is not evaporating, or else you will burn your pan dry during the night. Ask me how I know—three times!

4. At the 6-hour mark, uncover and begin to mash the chicken bones with a potato masher. Cover and continue to simmer. Repeat in 2 more hours and again if needed. You should be able to completely pulverize the bones.

5. At the end of cooking, remove the stockpot from the heat and strain off all solids into a clear glass bowl. Reserve soft, mushy solids to cool and feed to your favorite dog.

6. When fat rises to the top, skim it off with a large spoon. Reserve chicken fat for cooking, if you'd like. Since the bone broth contains all the minerals, it will naturally begin to gel. You may not even see much fat come to the surface, and that is fine.

7. Pour it into a 1-quart jar and transfer it to the refrigerator when adequately cooled. Watch your temperature and time. You do not want to allow the bone broth to be in the danger zone for bacteria growth. An hour should be long enough to cool the broth and guard against bacterial growth. You want to make sure it is completely cooled prior to refrigeration.

Tips: If the smell of the bones simmering is too strong for you, add a cut-up onion. You can simmer the bones in an oven set to 210°F, or even in a slow cooker turned to medium, as long as you can get a slow simmer. My mom will even put her slow cooker in the garage to keep the kitchen and the whole house from smelling like cooking chicken.

Chicken Stock

Chef Eddie
Yield: 6 quarts

The uses for chicken stock are varied. It is the root of all good and can be used to thin salad dressings without adding extra calories. When making salad dressing, use half the quantity of oil called for and replace the other half with this Chicken Stock recipe.

Ingredients:

7 quarts water
3 whole chickens, remove as much skin as you can
4 large yellow onions, unpeeled and quartered (leave the outer layers on for more depth of flavor)
4 celery stalks with leaves, cut into thirds
20 sprigs fresh parsley
15 sprigs fresh thyme
20 sprigs fresh dill
1 head garlic, unpeeled and cut in half crosswise
2 tablespoons kosher salt

Instructions:

1. Place all ingredients in a 16- to 20-quart stockpot.

2. Add water and bring to a boil. Simmer, uncovered, for 4 hours.

3. Strain entire contents of the pot through a colander and discard the solids.

4. Chill stock overnight. The next day, remove surface fat.

5. Use immediately or pack in containers and freeze for up to 3 months.

Phase 3 Variation: add 2 teaspoons whole black peppercorns and/or 6 carrots, unpeeled and halved.

Grilled Chicken with Peppered Artichokes and Parmesan

Chef Eddie
Serves: 4

When I was traveling and cooking, I would often end up in one of the business centers of the world. I looked at it as an opportunity to learn something new and stay on the cutting edge of the food world by visiting the showcase restaurants of the world's famous chefs. One of my favorites was Mario Battali.

The style of Italian food I grew up was very different than Mario's style of cooking. Pasta, heavy tomato sauce, meatballs and lots of garlic were the things I came to identify as Italian, and honestly, I didn't care for them. Even my just saying that makes me feel like I talked bad about the family, and I need to make a confession.

But at Mario's restaurants, I discovered lighter, very vibrant, and exciting combinations that, to me, were really unusual: combinations like artichokes and mint, chopped lemons and parmesan in salad, and real sardines with raisins and fennel. I learned that Italian food could be simple and delicious. This dish has certainly been influenced by him and his orange clogs.

Peppered Artichokes

Ingredients:
1 medium onion, cut into ¼-inch dice
3 garlic cloves mashed or diced
1 bay leaf
¼ cup extra-virgin olive oil
Sea salt
Red pepper flakes
24 artichokes hearts or bottoms, cleaned, cooked, and coarsely chopped
Fresh mint leaves for garnish (optional)
Parmigiano Reggiano cheese for shaving

Instructions:

1. Heat a sauté pan over medium-high heat with about 2 tablespoons of the olive oil. When the oil shimmers, add the onion and cook until soft, about 3 -5 minutes.

2. When the onion is ready, add artichokes, bay leaf, garlic, and salt, and toss until artichoke is cooked through. Note: the amount of time will depend on whether you're using fresh, frozen or jarred artichokes. Your purpose here is to get the artichokes cooked and blend all the flavors.

3. When artichokes are cooked through, remove from the heat and set aside. Sprinkle with red pepper flakes, drizzle on some more olive oil to coat, toss, and cool to room temperature. Let it rest for an hour or overnight in the refrigerator.

4. To serve, give it a taste and adjust the seasoning.

Simple Grilled Chicken

Ingredients:

1 garlic clove, minced
2 tablespoons extra-virgin olive oil or herbed oil of your choice
Sea salt, to taste
Creole or Santa Fe Seasoning Mix, to taste
4 free-range, organic chicken breasts

Instructions:

1. Place first four ingredients into a small bowl and mix well. Toss with the chicken breasts and let marinate for an hour or longer in the refrigerator.

2. Remove chicken from the refrigerator 15 minutes prior to cooking and set aside.

3. Preheat a grill to high heat and place the chicken breasts on the grill to sear, about 1 to 2 minutes per side. Turn the heat to medium-low and continue to cook for 6 to 8 minutes longer. Remove from the grill and let the chicken rest a few minutes prior to slicing.

To serve, plate a portion of chicken and artichokes, shave cheese on it, and sprinkle around some mint leaves, if desired.

Jumbo Lump Crab Salad or Hand Roll

Chef Eddie
Serves: 2 for main dish or 4 as an appetizer

I find as many ways as I can to eat crabmeat. This variation moves me outside my normal Cajun routine in a way that is totally agreeable.

Ingredients:

8 ounces jumbo lump crab (don't even think about using imitation crab)
⅓ cup cilantro or parsley, chopped
1 tablespoon raw agave
1 tablespoon extra-virgin olive oil
Sea salt, to taste
Cayenne pepper, to taste
¼ cup cucumber, peeled, seeded, and soaked in ice water for 15 minutes, then minced
Lemon juice, freshly pressed
4 toasted nori sheets

Instructions:

1. In a medium-size mixing bowl, gently fold together all ingredients, except lemon juice and nori sheets, being careful not to break up crab lumps.

2. Adjust seasonings and add lemon juice to taste.

3. Lay nori sheets out on the counter. Fill with crab salad and roll.

Tip: serve crab salad over greens.

Phase 3 Variation: Serve crab salad in ½ avocado. Or use Crab Ravigote to fill hand rolls.

Quinoa Cheesy Egg Muffins

Beth
Yield: 18

You can bag these muffins when cooled and keep them in the fridge for an anytime grab-and-go snack. Ivan and I like to take them on flights so we have something substantial to eat if we don't want the airline food.

Ingredients:

Extra-virgin olive oil for cooking
½ cup onions, diced
2 cloves garlic, minced
6 egg whites
1 cup raw goat's milk cheddar cheese, grated
¼ teaspoon sea salt
Cayenne pepper, dash (optional)
2 cups cooked sprouted quinoa, cooled

Instructions:

1. Preheat oven to 350°F.

2. Sauté the chopped onions in a little olive oil over medium-high heat and cook until translucent. Add the minced garlic and cook for 1 minute more, then allow to cool.

3. In a large bowl, whisk egg whites until slightly foamy. Add grated cheese, sautéed onions, and minced garlic to egg whites. Season with salt to taste (about ¼ teaspoon), and for a little zip, add a pinch of cayenne pepper, if you'd like.

4. Add cooled quinoa to the egg mixture and stir gently until all ingredients are combined.

5. Spoon the mixture into a paper-lined muffin tin and bake for 20–25 minutes or until lightly browned on top. Serve hot.

Tip: add some steamed spinach to the batter and stir it in before baking.

Phase 3 Variation: add sautéed tomatoes to the onions and garlic.

Southwestern Quinoa

Chef Eddie
Yield: ½ cup

There are a lot of things going on here that will make your mouth happy. The flavors are fresh, vibrant, and bold.

Ingredients:

½ cup sprouted quinoa, prepared
1 tablespoon red onion, finely diced
1 tablespoon extra-virgin olive oil
½ teaspoon lemon juice, freshly squeezed
⅛ teaspoon sea salt
½ cup cilantro, diced
½ teaspoon Santa Fe Seasoning Mix

Instructions:

1. In a medium-size mixing bowl, combine quinoa with onions and stir together.

2. Drizzle in olive oil and lemon juice and incorporate well.

3. Stir in sea salt, diced cilantro, and Santa Fe Seasoning Mix. Taste and adjust as needed. Serve warm or cold.

Phase 3 Variation: mix in 1 teaspoon jalapeño, seeds removed, stemmed, veined, and diced.

Spinach and Artichoke Soup

Chef Eddie
Yield: 1 quart

This is an old-line, New Orleans dish found in many of the great traditional restaurants here. Thickened up with a bit of creamy goat cheese, it makes a great dip, too. To liven it up further, add fresh shrimp or oysters.

Ingredients:

2 tablespoons extra-virgin olive oil
2 celery stalks, chopped
1 medium onion, chopped
One bag frozen artichoke hearts, thawed
Kosher salt, to taste
16 ounces Chicken Stock
1 cup spinach, packed fresh (about 1 ounce)
3 sprigs thyme, roughly chop leaves, discard stems
Lemon wedges

Instructions:

1. Heat olive oil in a large saucepan over medium heat.

2. Add celery, onion, and artichoke hearts. Season with salt to taste. Cook vegetables until just tender, about 4 minutes.

3. Add Chicken Stock and bring to a boil.

4. Cover, reduce heat to medium-low, and simmer until the artichoke hearts are tender, about 12 minutes.

5. Puree soup, a little at a time, in a blender until very smooth, adding spinach at the end. (Note: leave the plug out of the top of the blender or leave the top slightly askew while blending anything hot. If not, you will need to clean your ceiling.)

6. Return the puree to the same saucepan. Warm over low heat, adjust seasoning, and thin with additional Chicken Stock if soup is too thick.

7. Ladle soup into bowls. Scatter thyme leaves and squeeze a lemon wedge over each bowl of soup before serving.

Twenty-Seven

Complete Misner Plan Phase 3 Food List

VEGETABLES (ORGANIC)

Avocado
Artichoke
Asparagus
Bamboo shoots
Beets
Broccoli
Brussels sprouts
Cabbage (including bok choy and broccoli rabe)
Carrots
Cassava
Cauliflower
Celery
Cilantro
Cucumber
Eggplant
Garlic

Grape leaves

Green beans

Jerusalem artichoke

Jicama

Kale, including sea kale

Kohlrabi

Kombu

Leafy greens

Mushrooms

Nori

Okra

Olives (watch for preservatives)

Onions, yellow, white, red, all onion family vegetables, including scallions (green onions),

Shallots, leeks

Parsley, all types

Parsnips

Peas

Peppers, bell and hot

Potato (red, sweet, and yam)

Radish

Rhubarb

Rutabaga

Sprouts

Summer squash (yellow, Italian, Mexican gray)

Tomatoes, all types (cooked fresh tomatoes are best for sauces)

Turnips

Water chestnut

Watercress

Winter squash (acorn, butternut, pumpkin, and spaghetti)

Zucchini

Lacto-fermented vegetables are permitted, such as sauerkraut, kimchi, and miso

No corn, unless is it certified GMO-free

No soybeans, unless organic, non-GMO, and fermented, as in miso, in very small quantities

WHOLE GRAINS (ORGANIC)

Cooked from sprouted grains until chewy, not crunchy or soggy:

Amaranth

Barley

Brown rice (California or Texas)

Buckwheat

Einkorn

Oatmeal, specified gluten-free

Kamut

Millet

Quinoa

Teff

Gluten-free pasta is fine, in limited quantities and frequency

No white rice of any type, including risotto

No couscous or farro

Consume gluten grains (barley, einkorn, kamut, and spelt) in limited quantities and frequencies

SEASONINGS AND HERBS (ORGANIC)

Anise

Basil

Bay leaves

Cardamom

Cayenne and red pepper flakes

Cilantro, fresh or dry

Cinnamon

Curcumin

Dill

Garlic, dry powdered

Ginger (dry or peeled and freshly grated)

Horseradish, freshly grated

Italian seasoning

Mint

Mustard (dry powdered)

Oregano, fresh or dry

Parsley, fresh or dry

Pepper, fresh cracked (red, green, black)

Rosemary, fresh or dry

Saffron

Sea salt

Thyme

Turmeric

Vanilla bean (not extract)

Sweeten with raw organic honey, raw organic coconut nectar, or raw organic maguey sap

No stevia (unless you grow your own stevia plant and use the leaves, dried or fresh, or you are able to get stevia leaf)

No sugars of any kind (including raw, brown, sucrose, fructose, xylitol, and beet)

If you have any problems with inflammation: no vinegars or foods containing, or having been marinated in, vinegar

LEGUMES/PULSES (ORGANIC)

Beans should be soaked/germinated before cooking:

Adzuki beans

Black beans

Black-eyed peas

Broad (or fava) beans

Butter beans

Cannellini beans

Garbanzo beans

Green split peas, dried

Lentil beans

Lima beans

Kidney beans

Mung beans

Navy beans

Pinto beans

Red beans

White beans

No edamame/soybeans, unless non-GMO fermented soy, such as miso

FRUITS (ORGANIC)

Fruits should be eaten fresh or dried with no preservatives, added sugars, or artificial colors:

Apples

Apricots

Bananas

Berries

Black cherries

Coconut

Dates

Dragon fruit

Figs

Grapes

Grapefruit

Guavas

Jujubes

Kiwis

Kumquats

Lemons

Loquats

Mangoes

Melons

Nectarines

Oranges (all types)

Papayas

Peaches

Pears

Persimmons

Pineapples

Plums

Pomegranates

Pomelos

Raisins
Star fruit
Tangerines

OILS (ORGANIC)
These oils should be used cold, added to foods after cooking:
Butternut squash seed oil
Citrus oils (used by the drop for flavoring)
Flaxseed oil
Nut oils, such as sesame, walnut, hazelnut
Pumpkin seed oil
Safflower oil

These oils may be used cold *and* for cooking:
Coconut oil
Ghee
Grapeseed oil
Olive oil, extra-virgin, fresh press
Tea seed oil
No canola oil
No peanut oil
No lard
No butter (except ghee)

BEVERAGES (ORGANIC)
Clean, purified, alkaline water
Green tea
Herbal tea with no added natural flavors
Freshly juiced fruit and vegetable juices (drink within the first 10 minutes of juicing for maximum nutrition)

ANIMAL PROTEIN
Cheese, goat's milk or sheep's milk, with no mold inhibitors (e.g., natamycin), hard cheeses in small quantities, such as Parmesan, Asiago, and Romano (made with cow's milk), with no mold inhibitors, Mizithra cheese (goat's or sheep's milk) with no mold inhibitors

Eggs, organic, pasture raised when possible with 1 yolk per 3 whites

Poultry, antibiotic- and hormone-free, about once every 2 weeks

Chicken
Turkey

Meats (red)
Antibiotic- and hormone-free lamb (about once every 2 weeks)
Wild meats: venison, elk, bison, and ostrich (about once every 2 weeks)
Grass-fed, grass-finished beef (about once every 3 weeks to 1 month)

Seafood (should be wild caught and not farmed)

Cod
Flounder
Haddock
Lobster
Salmon
Scallops
Shrimp
White fish

Yogurt, plain, organic, made from goat's or sheep's milk when possible, and only if you have no inflammatory conditions

RAW NUTS (ORGANIC)
Unless otherwise indicated below, raw nuts should be soaked in warm water for a minimum of 7 hours, or overnight, and then dried in a low-heat oven on 150°F for 12–24 hours, until completely dried:
Almonds
Brazil nuts (limit to 2 per day)
Cashews (soak only 2 hours and dry at 200°F for 12–24 hours)
Hazelnuts/Filberts
Macadamia nuts (soak only 4 hours and dry at 150°F for 12–24 hours)

Pecans
Pine nuts (do not need to be soaked)
Pistachios (do not need to be soaked)
Walnuts
No dry roasted nuts
No peanuts

SEEDS/NIBS (ORGANIC)

Should be eaten raw, unless indicated otherwise:
Cacao
Carob
Chia
Flax (grind freshly before use)
Hemp (grind freshly before use)
Poppy
Pumpkin (may be roasted at a low temperature)
Sesame
Squash (may be roasted at a low temperature)
Sunflower
Watermelon
Wild Rice

MILK ALTERNATIVES (ORGANIC)

It is best to make these milk alternatives yourself. Commercially prepared milk alternatives usually contain many other added ingredients, such as carrageenan and sugar, as well as preservatives. Remember to use germinated nuts/grains for these milk alternatives.
Almond milk
Brown rice milk
Coconut milk
Hazelnut milk
Hemp milk
No soy milk

Phase 3 Supplement Schedule

WITH MEALS
2 Premier Digest
1 Premier Clay
1 Premier Probiotics

To maintain body detoxification during Phase 3, enjoy one Medi-Clay-FX and one Medi-Body Bath on alternating weeks.

Twenty-Eight

PHASE 3 RECIPES

Baba Ghanoush

Chef Eddie
Serves: 4

I love baba ghanoush. It is very versatile. You can serve it as a side dish with any meats or fish that you cook. Use this certainly as a dip with your root chips, or use it like a mayonnaise spread on a sandwich.

Ingredients:
1 pound purple, Japanese, green, or white eggplants
1 clove garlic, minced
½ teaspoon sea salt
¼ teaspoon cayenne pepper
⅛ teaspoon white pepper, ground
¼ cup flat-leaf parsley, finely chopped, plus more for garnish
2 tablespoons Homemade Nut Butter, cashew
2 tablespoons lemon juice

Instructions:

1. Preheat oven to 450°F.

2. Prick eggplant with a fork and place on a cookie sheet lined with foil. Don't skip that part. Eggplant skin is not porous. If you put it in the oven without pricking it, you will hear a loud thump, which will be an eggplant explosion all over your oven. Ask me how I know.

3. Bake eggplant until it is soft inside, about 20 minutes. Alternately, you can grill eggplant over a gas grill or over the burner on your gas stove, rotating until skin is completely charred, about 10 minutes. Let eggplant cool. This will add a touch of smokiness and a bit of depth to it.

4. Cut eggplant in half lengthwise, drain off liquid, and scoop pulp into food processor. Process eggplant until smooth and transfer to a medium-size bowl.

5. On a cutting board, work garlic and ¼ teaspoon salt together with the flat side of a knife until it forms a paste. Adding sea salt to the garlic helps keep chopped garlic from sticking to the knife blade.

6. Add garlic mixture to the eggplant and stir together.

7. Add salt and cayenne and ground white pepper to taste.

8. Stir in parsley, cashew butter, and lemon juice. Season with more salt, to taste. Adjust lemon juice to taste.

9. Garnish with additional parsley, a few olives, and serve with vegetable root chips for dipping.

Tip: this would be good with Veggie Meatballs, as well!

Baked Egg Muffins

Chef Eddie
Yield: 6

Great for grab-and-go, you can eat these as they come out of the oven, or reheat them quickly.

Ingredients:

7 eggs
3 ounces sparkling water or orange juice
¼ teaspoon fine sea salt
⅛ teaspoon cayenne pepper
Ghee or extra-virgin olive oil, for cooking

Instructions:

1. Preheat oven to 350°F.

2. Combine all the ingredients in a mixing bowl, blend with an immersion blender or whisk strongly.

3. Coat a muffin tin with ghee or olive oil. Using a 3-ounce ladle, fill each of 6 cups in the muffin tin with the egg mixture. Bake for approximately 15 minutes or until the egg mixture is firm.

4. Remove from the oven and serve.

Tip: The addition of the sparking water will also allow these to be frozen and used later as a grab-and-go. Simply let them cool after removing from the oven and then wrap them in clear wrap or store in an airtight container and freeze. Remove them from the freezer the night before and defrost in the fridge overnight. Reheat in a 300°F oven for 10 minutes.

Black Beans

Chef Eddie
Serves: 4

I am addicted to this dish, and it is a staple in my house. The beans are so good and so bright that they add excitement to whatever dish you use them in. They go great alongside chicken or fish. You can make a mean black bean dip with them, or you can use them for black bean cakes and top with shrimp and Cashew Cream. Another great aspect of this dish is you can sauté your vegetables and then just throw it all in a slow cooker, go to work, and come home to a wonderful meal. I love these things.

Ingredients:

1 pound dried black beans, soaked overnight in water to cover
1 tablespoon extra-virgin olive oil
1 large onion, chopped
2 tablespoons garlic, minced
2 poblano peppers, chopped
2 tablespoons Santa Fe Seasoning Mix
1 tablespoon sea salt
2 quarts Chicken Stock
¼ teaspoon cayenne pepper, optional
¼ teaspoon cumin, optional
1 bunch cilantro, coarsely chopped
Juice of one lime, freshly squeezed

Instructions:

1. Drain and rinse the beans.

2. Heat oil in a large skillet over medium-high heat. When the oil is hot, add onions, garlic, and poblano and sauté, stirring occasionally for 4 minutes. You want the onions to start browning nicely.

3. Add beans, Santa Fe Seasoning Mix, and sea salt to the pan and sauté for 2 minutes. Add stock, bring to a boil, lower the heat, then simmer for 50–60 minutes, or until the beans are tender. Beans vary in cooking time, so be patient.

4. After the beans have cooked for about 30 minutes, give them a taste. You are looking for some flavors here. The beans will still be very firm, but you should be able to taste the chili and cumin from the Santa Fe Seasoning, and the salt should be in balance. If you want some more heat, add cayenne pepper. If it lacks some depth or some "southwestern-ness," add cumin or cayenne *and* cumin. If you think it needs salt, you can add a little, but don't overdo it. The lime juice at the end may take care of that. The point is, unless beans are in a slow cooker, adjust as you go.

5. Keep simmering, making sure there is enough stock to just slightly cover the beans. When the beans are tender, stir in cayenne pepper, cilantro, and lime juice and simmer for about 5 minutes longer. Taste again and make your final adjustments. Beans should rich, bright, and have enough heat and flavor to make your mouth dance.

6. Remove from the heat. Serve immediately.

Tip: If the beans are a little runny, take your immersion blender and pulse 3 or 4 times. Let the beans cook about 10 minutes more, and that should give you the consistency you are looking for.

This dish is spectacular topped with a little Santa Fe Crema and diced red onion if you have it.

Black-Eyed Pea Jambalaya

Chef Eddie
Serves: 4

Black-eyed peas are a really underused ingredient. I first discovered how to use them when I had company coming over and reached into my pantry for some chickpeas, only to find out I didn't have them. I did have a few pounds of black-eyed peas, however. Well, what to do? I cooked them and turned them into a black-eyed pea relish that was a big hit, and I realized these things are really good, particularly in winter. Nice and hearty with a good flavor base. I am sure you will be using these more after you try this dish.

Ingredients:

2 tablespoons extra-virgin olive oil
1 pound yellow onion, chopped
1 poblano pepper, seeded and chopped
2 stalks celery, chopped
12 ounces Italian Sausage, chicken version
1 pound black-eyed peas, fresh or dried
3 bay leaves
Sea salt, to taste
Cayenne pepper, to taste
1 quart Chicken Stock (if using dried peas, you may need 2 quarts)
3 cups pulled grass-fed, grass-finished beef shoulder, pulled organic chicken, or chopped firm mushrooms

Instructions:

1. Heat olive oil in large 4- to 5-quart pot, preferably cast iron, over medium-high heat until shimmering. Add onions, peppers, and celery and reduce heat to medium-high. Sauté until the vegetables begin to brown, about 10 minutes. If you are using sausage, add it to the vegetables at this point.

2. Add peas and bay leaves and continue to cook for about 7 minutes. The bay leaves should make the kitchen very fragrant. If you are using pulled beef, chicken, or mushrooms, add it at this point.

3. Every minute or so, while the vegetables are cooking, scrape the bottom of the pot to loosen up the browned bits. This is where the flavor is. After the vegetables are nicely cooked, add the stock and clear the bottom of the pot once more.

4. Reduce heat to a simmer and cook until peas are soft or the texture you like. Taste as they cook and adjust the seasonings as you like. If it tastes a little flat, add some sea salt. If it needs heat, add peppers. As the peas near completion, they will go from nearly done to stuck-to-the-bottom-and-burned very quickly. Keep an eye on them.

Tip: you can use Vegetable Stock, if you like.

Italian Sausage

Chef Eddie
Yield: 12 small patties

Discovering the Misner Plan will open your eyes to how many things we have stopped making from scratch in our own kitchens. Sausage is one of them, and it is beyond simple to make a flavorful, healthy sausage you can enjoy in a wide range of other dishes. You get to use the fresh meat and spices of your choice, all while avoiding the undesirables: preservatives, chemical additives, and sugar. Including fruits, both fresh and dried, gives texture and sweetness that complement the heat from your seasonings. You will return to this recipe several times throughout the Misner Plan cookbook, because we use it as a key component of several other dishes.

Ingredients:
1 pound ground chicken (or try ground turkey, lamb, beef, venison, or even a combination)
1 teaspoon rubbed sage
1 teaspoon thyme
¼ teaspoon salt
¼ teaspoon cayenne
½ teaspoon red pepper flakes
¼ teaspoon cloves, ground
1 teaspoon cinnamon
¼ teaspoon nutmeg
1 teaspoon fennel seeds
1 small pear or apple, cored and finely diced
2 tablespoons dried cranberries or cherries (no added sugar or coloring), chopped
Coconut oil for sautéing

Instructions:
1. In a large bowl, combine all ingredients until well blended, using a large spoon, or like Gram did, with her hands.

2. Form mixture into 12 small patties.

3. Sauté patties in a large skillet over medium heat with a small amount of oil for 2–3 minutes per side, or until cooked through. Serve hot.

Caesar Salad

Beth

Serves: 4

The great thing about the Misner Plan is that you can still eat traditional foods, like this great Caesar Salad. We aren't about restricting foods; we are all about replacing ingredients that don't serve our bodies well. Enjoy.

Ingredients:

2 full heads Romaine lettuce leaves
Eddie's Caesar Dressing
½ cup Parmesan cheese, freshly grated

Instructions:

1. Tear Romaine lettuce leaves in bite-size pieces into a mixing bowl.

2. Add Eddie's Caesar Dressing to coat and finish with Parmesan cheese.

Variations: top with grilled chicken, grilled or baked salmon, or other seafood.

Cajun Slaw

Chef Eddie
Serves: 4 as a small salad or 8 as a condiment, as on fish tacos or black beans

This slaw makes a great topping for fish, or include it in fish tacos for a fresh Baja taste.

Ingredients:

2 cups white cabbage, shredded
2 cups red cabbage, shredded
½ pound assorted greens (such as mustard greens, chard, or spinach) trimmed, washed, and shredded (about 2 cups)
1 cup red onions, thinly sliced
1 cup scallion (green onion) tops, chopped
½ cup parsley leaves, chopped
1¼ cups homemade mayonnaise
¼ cup Creole or whole-grain mustard (find one with apple cider vinegar)
1 teaspoon sea salt
¼ teaspoon black pepper, freshly ground
¼ teaspoon cayenne pepper
1 teaspoon maguey sap or coconut nectar

Instructions:

1. Combine ingredients in a large mixing bowl and toss well to incorporate.

2. Enjoy as a main dish or a salad before a larger meal.

Cashew Crusted Chicken Fingers

Chef Eddie
Serves: 4

My kids were the taste testers for these chicken fingers. The crumbs on the bottom of the serving platter gave testimony to their opinion. Pretty sure they will be asking for these again and again.

Ingredients:

1 pound free-range chicken fingers
½ cup gluten-free flour blend
2 tablespoons Santa Fe Seasoning Mix
1 large egg
¾ cup almond milk
2 cups finely chopped (in food processor) cashew nuts
Olive oil, for cooking

Instructions:

1. Sprinkle chicken fingers on both sides with some of the Santa Fe Seasoning Mix.

2. In a bowl, combine flour with remaining seasoning mix.

3. In another bowl, beat the egg together with the milk.

4. Place chopped cashew nuts in a third bowl.

5. Dredge chicken in the seasoned flour, then the egg wash, then the cashew nuts, pressing the nuts thickly all over on the chicken. Set aside.

6. Heat enough oil to cover the bottom of the skillet you will be using and come ¼ inch up the side on medium-high heat until the oil begins to shimmer, or you can see some heat rising from the pan. Sauté chicken until golden, for about 5 minutes on each side, taking care not to burn cashews.

7. Transfer cooked chicken fingers to a serving platter and serve with Poblano Sauce, other favorite Misner Plan sauce, or any of our Olive Oil Mayos.

Tip: If the fingers are thick, it may be better to brown the chicken in the skillet and then transfer the chicken to a 350° oven to finish. If you are serving a larger group, this would be the way to do it, to avoid doing batches on the run.

Chicken and Sausage Gumbo

Chef Eddie
Serves: 8

In my part of the world, this is a regular, everyday dish. Funny thing is people come from all over the world to New Orleans to get it. I made this version Misner Plan friendly, but frankly, I have been eating and serving it this way for years, and people love it.

Ingredients:

Extra-virgin olive oil for cooking
1⅓ cups Italian Sausage (chicken version), diced
1 poblano pepper, diced
1 yellow pepper, diced
1 large yellow onion, diced
2 stalks celery, diced
1⅓ tablespoons Creole Seasoning Mix
1 teaspoon sea salt
1 roasted chicken, skinned (see tips below)
½ teaspoon cayenne pepper
4 bay leaves
2 teaspoons garlic, minced
2 quarts Chicken Stock
1 stalk thyme
1 stalk oregano
4 cups brown rice, cooked
4 scallions, chopped

Instructions:

1. In a 6-quart cast-iron stockpot (Dutch oven), cover the bottom with just enough olive oil to make it moist, about 2 tablespoons. For about 2 minutes, heat the pot over high heat until the oil starts to shimmer or you see steam starting to rise.

2. Place diced sausage in the pot and sauté until the sausage is browned, about 2 minutes.

3. Place peppers, onion, and celery, into the pot. Add 1 teaspoon of Creole Seasoning Mix and sea salt. Reduce heat to medium high and sauté until most of the vegetables are golden brown (about 10 minutes). Be sure to scrape the bottom of the pot every couple of minutes while vegetables are cooking to get up caramelized brown bits on the bottom. These bits are full of flavor, and we don't want them to burn.

4. At this point you should see what looks like the beginnings of a nice, rich, dark-colored juice at the bottom of the pot. Add chicken, remaining Creole Seasoning Mix, cayenne pepper, bay leaves, and garlic. Stir, scraping bottom of pot for 1 more minute.

5. Turn heat to high, add about 8 ounces of Chicken Stock to the pot, scrape and deglaze the bottom of the pot. You will definitely see a very nicely colored juice in the bottom at this point. You will be tempted, but don't eat it.

6. Add remainder of Chicken Stock, thyme, and oregano, and bring to a slow boil. Reduce heat and simmer for 1 hour. Be sure to taste and adjust seasonings along the way.

7. To serve, put ½ cup cooked brown rice in the bottom of soup bowl, ladle in gumbo, and garnish each bowl with some chopped scallions.

Note: in South Louisiana it is normal to have chicken or meat bones in a rustic soup like this. Many a gumbo has been made with leftover pieces of chicken, fish, pork, or you name it. The bones will give a depth of flavor and richness to the dish, so go ahead and throw that rotisserie chicken in there. The meat will also fall right off the bone, so you won't have to handle the hot bones to eat it.

If having chicken bones in your dish is not your thing, then debone the chicken and put the pulled meat into the soup. Wrap the bones in cheesecloth, and put them back into the pot. When the soup is done, discard the cheesecloth, and off you go.

This is also a little different gumbo than traditional gumbo, as there is no roux. A roux is a dark, cooked mixture of flour and oil used to thicken the gumbo, and it is also the basis for many a Cajun dish. In fact, they may make me move when they find out there is no roux in this gumbo. This will save a ton of calories, though, and still result in a delicious soup.

Chickpea (Garbanzo Beans) Recipe

Chef Eddie
Yield: about 3 quarts

A classic ingredient among vegetarians and vegans is beans. Black, red, white—you name it, they use it. One bean that gets underused for the most part is chickpeas (or garbanzo beans). While their use in hummus is widely known, just having them stand alone is rarely seen in the restaurant world or on family tables. It's a shame, really, because these things are good. So let's change that, starting now. This recipe is basic, but the beans can be seasoned a number of ways—from Creole and Cajun to Southwest and Indian. You're going to love having them.

Ingredients:

1 pound chickpeas, soaked overnight
Extra-virgin olive oil for cooking chickpeas
1 poblano pepper, diced
1 large yellow onion, diced
2 stalks celery, diced
1 yellow pepper, diced
2 tablespoons garlic, minced
1 teaspoon sea salt
½ teaspoon cayenne pepper
8 cups Chicken Stock
3 bay leaves

Instructions:

1. Soak the garbanzo beans overnight in the refrigerator with water that is at least 3 times the volume of the beans.

2. Cover the bottom of a 6-quart cast-iron pot (Dutch oven) with a little olive oil, about 2 tablespoons, and heat over high heat. When the oil starts to shimmer or you see a bit of steam rising from the pan, place all vegetables into the pot, add a little sea salt and pepper, reduce the heat to medium-high, and sauté. Cook, scraping the bottom of the pot periodically,

until the vegetables turn a nice golden brown, about 7 minutes. If your pot looks a little dry, splash in just a bit more oil.

3. Add the chickpeas, remainder of sea salt, pepper, and bay leaves and continue to sauté everything together for another 3 minutes, continually scraping the bottom every minute or so.

4. Add enough Chicken Stock to cover the mixture by an inch or so and bring to a slow boil. Then reduce heat to low and simmer.

5. Simmer for about 1½ to 2 hours, occasionally tasting and adjusting seasoning, making sure beans are just slightly covered by stock until they are soft.

Tip: depending on how you intend to use beans, try them with some Creole Seasoning Mix.

Cool Avocado Soup

Chef Eddie
Serves: 2

This soup is delicious as is, but some alternative spices to add could be chili powder and cumin, or for an Indian accent, curry-like spices, such as garam masala or curry powder, will be perfect.

Ingredients:

1 Haas avocado
1 cucumber, seeded and cubed
¼ cup Greek yogurt, goat's or sheep's milk
1 cup cold water
Half a lime, juiced
1 clove garlic
1 tablespoon extra-virgin olive oil
¼ bunch cilantro
Substantial pinch of sea salt
¼ teaspoon cayenne

Instructions:

1. Place all ingredients in a Vitamix or blender on medium-high speed. Puree until smooth. Taste for seasoning. Adjust as necessary.

2. Serve in small bowls and garnish as below. Eat immediately.

Tip: possible garnishes for this dish are diced red onion, jalapeño, cilantro, a dollop of Greek yogurt, or some chopped tomato.

Crab Ravigote

Chef Eddie
Serves: 4

Although ravigote is of French origin, this is a New Orleans favorite found in many of the old-line, famous restaurants. It is probably a little too traditional for a lot of new restaurant menus, but it is off-the-page good and extremely versatile. You can serve it with a green salad, scoop it into half an avocado, tuck it in a sushi-style hand roll, or as a dip with celery root chips.

No matter how you serve it, the star of the show is the crabmeat. Use jumbo lump blue crab or big pieces of Dungeness crab, and this is a surefire winner for guests or just for you.

Ingredients:
½ cup Olive Oil Mayonnaise
2 teaspoons Amy's brand organic Dijon mustard made with apple cider vinegar
2 teaspoons lemon juice, freshly squeezed
½ teaspoon garlic, minced
¼ teaspoon cayenne pepper
¼ teaspoon sea salt
2 tablespoons scallions, chopped
¼ cup tomatoes, seeded, diced small
1 tablespoon shallots, minced
1 tablespoon fresh parsley, chopped
1 pound jumbo lump or lump crabmeat, picked over for shells and cartilage

Instructions:
1. Whisk Olive Oil Mayonnaise, mustard, lemon juice, garlic, cayenne pepper, and sea salt in the bottom of a medium bowl. Give it a taste. The adjustments you need will likely come by stepping up the mustard, heat, or lemon juice. Adjust until you love it and then go to the next step.

2. Fold in scallions, tomatoes, shallots, and parsley. Gently fold in crabmeat, turning to gently coat with dressing and being careful not to break up the lumps.

3. Adjust seasoning, to taste, and serve.

Crawfish Étouffée

Chef Eddie
Serves: 4

"First you got to make a good roux." In Cajun cooking, many recipes start with this verbiage. A good roux is the basis for a lot of things. In our version we use gluten-free or garbanzo flour, but use whatever one you like. Just be careful not to burn it, and don't stop stirring.

Ingredients:

½ cup ghee
½ cup garbanzo or other gluten-free flour
1 tablespoon + 1 teaspoon Creole Seasoning Mix
1 small red, yellow, or orange pepper, diced
1 large yellow onion, diced small
3 celery stalks, diced
32 ounces organic Fumet de Poisson (or Chicken Stock, if that's what you have)
3 bay leaves
1 teaspoon oregano
1 teaspoon thyme
1 teaspoon cayenne pepper
1 pound crawfish tails or small shrimp
½ teaspoon lemon juice
2 scallions, chopped

Instructions:

1. In 5-quart cast iron pot, melt ghee over medium heat until it's good and hot. Add garbanzo flour a little at a time, stirring consistently with a whisk until dark brown, about 12 minutes.

2. Add Creole Seasoning Mix, diced pepper, onion, and celery to roux in the pot. Stir and cook approximately 5 minutes, until vegetables are mostly cooked.

3. Add stock, bay leaves, 1 teaspoon sea salt, oregano, thyme, and cayenne pepper. Cook until flour flavor is gone, about 20–30 minutes. Unlike traditional flours, there will likely still

be a bit of the flour flavor present after the simmering. For example, you will taste a hint of garbanzo bean in the dish, but not the flour taste.

4. Remove bay leaves.

5. Put crawfish tails into a bowl and add ½ teaspoon Creole Seasoning Mix, to taste. Turn off heat and add crawfish tails to the étouffée. Taste and adjust seasonings. Note: if using shrimp, add them to the hot étouffée for 7 minutes to cook them while it is still simmering.

6. Serve over brown rice, sprinkle with some chopped scallions and lemon juice.

Creole Crab Cakes

Chef Eddie
Serves: 4–6

Crab cakes made with generous lumps of delicious, fresh crabmeat are a real treat. Fortunately for me, Louisiana has an abundance of crab both from the brackish waters of Lake Pontchartrain and from the slightly less brackish bays and bayous of the lower coastal areas. In fact, it is still common to see people with crab nets fishing right off the seawall of the lake, just as I did growing up.

Crab is also quite versatile. Soft shell crabs, spicy boiled crabs, gumbo crabs, stuffed crabs, crab ravigote—you can see how easy it is to get captivated by them and the number of ways they can be used. These crab cakes are great served with Creole Tartar Sauce or topped with a poached egg for Sunday brunch. If you have trouble getting good crabmeat, don't hesitate to substitute chopped shrimp or crayfish tails in place of the crab.

Crab Cake Base

Ingredients:
2 tablespoons extra-virgin olive oil
1½ cups yellow onions, diced small
½ cup celery, diced small
⅓ cup red bell peppers, diced small
⅓ cup yellow bell peppers, diced small
Sea salt, to taste
Pinch Creole Seasoning Mix
1 tablespoon garlic, minced
1 pound lump crabmeat, cleaned and picked over for shells and cartilage
¼ cup scallions, chopped
¼ to ½ cup Parmigiano Reggiano cheese, grated
2 tablespoons parsley leaves, finely chopped

3 tablespoons Creole mustard or brown, whole-grain mustard (made with apple cider vinegar)
2 tablespoons lemon juice, freshly squeezed

Instructions:

1. Heat the olive oil in a medium-size sauté pan over medium heat. Add the onions, celery, and peppers; season with salt and a pinch of Creole Seasoning Mix; and sauté for 5 minutes. Add the garlic and continue to sauté for 2 minutes. Remove the pan from the heat and cool for 5 minutes. Set aside in small bowl.

2. In a medium-size mixing bowl, combine crabmeat, scallions, grated cheese, parsley, Creole mustard, and lemon juice. Mix to incorporate. Taste it. The mixture should taste really good at this point. If you think it needs more mustard or cheese or seasoning, add it until you love the taste. Then you're ready to move on.

3. Set the mixture aside.

Creole Mayonnaise

Ingredients:

1 cup Olive Oil Mayonnaise
Sea salt, to taste
Black pepper, to taste
½ teaspoon Vegan Worcestershire Sauce
¼ teaspoon Portuguese Hot Pepper Sauce

Instructions:

1. Season Olive Oil Mayonnaise with salt and pepper to taste, add Vegan Worcestershire Sauce and Portuguese Hot Sauce, and then process the mixture to incorporate.

2. Taste, adjust seasonings until you love it.

Assemble Crab Cakes

Ingredients:
½ cup Creole Mayonnaise
¾ cups fine, gluten-free bread crumbs
¼ cup gluten-free flour blend
3 teaspoons Creole Seasoning Mix
Pinch of sea salt
1 egg
1 tablespoon water
¾ cups gluten-free panko

Instructions:
1. Fold the cooled, sautéed vegetables into the crab mixture along with the Creole Mayonnaise and bread crumbs. Mix gently but thoroughly, trying to leave the crab lumps intact.

2. In a shallow bowl, season the flour with 1 teaspoon of the Creole Seasoning Mix and a pinch of sea salt. In another bowl, whisk the remaining egg with the water to make an egg wash. Finally in another bowl, combine the panko and 1 teaspoon Creole Seasoning Mix.

3. Divide the filling into ⅓-cup balls or the portion size you are looking for. Taste it—you know the drill. If you love it, form the balls into patties, about 1 inch thick.

4. Dredge the cakes in the seasoned flour and shake off the excess. Dip the cakes in the egg wash, letting the excess egg wash drip off. Dredge the cakes in the seasoned panko, covering the cakes completely. Prepare them all and set them aside.

5. Using an olive oil spray-bottle mister, spray crab cakes on each side and place them on a baking rack. Place the rack in a heated oven and cook until cakes are nicely browned, the coating is crunchy, and the cakes are heated through, about 15 minutes. Season the cakes with the remaining Creole Seasoning Mix.

6. Serve Creole Crab Cakes with a dollop of Creole Mayonnaise, and sit back to watch your guests enjoy this dish.

Tip: As a fancy serving option, press the mixture into a cupcake pan. They will cook a bit faster, but you'll have the dimple in the middle to put a great filling, like guacamole or a poached egg yolk.

Crispy Chickpeas

Chef Eddie
Yield: 2 cups

This is a tasty snack food that can substitute for popcorn or be used in place of croutons in any salad dishes. You'll be surprised at how filling they are.

Ingredients:

2 cups chickpeas, cooked
1–2 teaspoons extra-virgin olive oil, or olive oil spray-bottle mister
¼ teaspoon salt
¼ teaspoon cayenne pepper
¼ teaspoon paprika
¼ teaspoon garlic powder

Instructions:

1. Preheat oven to 425°F.

2. Place chickpeas on a paper towel and pat completely dry. Remove any loose skins.

3. Place on a baking sheet and mist with olive oil. Roll around to coat. Sprinkle with seasonings of your choice and toss well to coat. Make sure chickpeas are in a single layer.

4. Bake for 15 minutes, toss well, and flip, then bake for about 15 minutes. Let them cool and eat.

Curried Cauliflower

Chef Eddie
Serves: 4

Anything you can do to make cauliflower more interesting is fine with me. Roasting and seasoning with the variety of spices can make an otherwise bland vegetable belong on the plate.

Ingredients:

3 tablespoons coconut oil, melted
½ teaspoon lemon zest
1 tablespoon curry powder or garam masala
1 teaspoon garlic powder
½ teaspoon turmeric
1 head of cauliflower florets
½ cup yogurt, goat's or sheep's milk
Sea salt and pepper, to taste

Instructions:

1. Preheat oven to 375°F.

2. Line a baking sheet with parchment paper.

3. In a large bowl, mix melted coconut oil and spices (reserve the sea salt and pepper), then add cauliflower florets and stir until all florets are coated.

4. Spread cauliflower onto a prepared baking sheet and bake for 40–45 minutes. Watch for a light, golden brown color.

5. Mix yogurt with sea salt and cracked pepper to taste and finish by tossing with cooked cauliflower.

Earl Grey Marinated Chicken

Chef Eddie
Serves: 4

A good friend and customer of mine came to me once and wanted a dish similar to what he had found in a restaurant. It was a tea-marinated fish, but he thought that chicken would be good as well. I researched the dish and found it was done with oolong tea. I tried it, and it tasted like—nothing.

I kept working it until we came upon good old Earl Grey tea. This provided the boldness needed for the heavier chicken, and it was a hit. I marinated it overnight and then cooked it in a cast-iron skillet as outlined below. The color was beautiful, and the tea flavor was just right.

You may need to adjust the amount of tea used for marinating, depending on its strength. Different brands generate different flavor profiles. Be sure there is a good covering of tea on the chicken.

Ingredients:
¼ cup dry white wine
2 tablespoons raw blue agave
1 tablespoon Bragg's Liquid Aminos
3 tablespoons Earl Grey tea leaves
½ lemon, freshly squeezed
3 tablespoons extra-virgin olive oil
4 chicken breasts, boneless and skinless

Instructions:
1. Preheat oven to 350°F.

2. In a medium-size bowl, combine wine, agave, Bragg's Liquid Aminos, tea leaves, lemon juice, and olive oil. Mix well. Pour marinade into a gallon-size resealable storage bag, and then add chicken, shake, and refrigerate overnight.

3. The next day, remove the chicken from the marinade. Strain the marinade and set liquid aside. Count out the tea leaves to put over the pieces of chicken as they are cooking.

4. Put about 3 tablespoons of reserved marinade into a cast-iron skillet. Heat over medium-high heat until the liquid is hot and looks to be shimmering slightly. Add chicken, with the tea leaves on top of each piece, and cook for a few minutes on each side until chicken is well colored.

5. Add a little more marinade to the top of each breast (about 1 teaspoon each), place the whole skillet in the oven, and cook until breasts are done, about 10 minutes.

6. Serve with a grains dish and vegetable side for a delightful meal.

Eggplant Chips

Chef Eddie
Yield: 3 cups

You are going to want to serve these chips with a dressing, rather than a dip, as they will be on the thin side and will be delicate.

Ingredients:

1 large eggplant
Coconut oil in a pump-spray mister, for cooking
Sea salt
Seasoning Mix of choice

Instructions:

1. Preheat oven to 400°F.

2. Use a mandoline or knife to slice eggplant into thin chips, about 1/16-inch thick. Place slices on a parchment-lined half-sheet pan. Excessively salt the slices, and let them sit for about 15 minutes.

3. Place slices in a bowl and rinse well. Dry with paper towels by squeezing out as much moisture as possible.

4. Place a drying rack on a half-sheet pan, place chips on rack, and spray with coconut oil, making sure not to soak them too much. Flip and spray the other side.

5. Sprinkle with Seasoning Mix of your choice.

6. Place in oven for about 10 minutes. Flip each chip over, then bake for another 10 minutes, or until they're golden brown.

7. Move chips from pan to a cooling rack. They will crisp up more as they cool.

Firecracker Soup

Beth Misner
Serves: 2

When you are hungry for a full-flavored, spicy soup, Firecracker Soup is for you!

Ingredients:

¼ medium white onion, diced
2 large unpeeled carrots, grated
1 fairly large sweet potato, peeled and chopped into cubes
Chicken Bone Broth, to cover
¼ teaspoon sea salt
⅛ teaspoon cumin
⅛ teaspoon turmeric
1 teaspoon fresh ginger, grated
Sprinkle paprika
Dash onion powder
Black pepper, freshly ground, to taste
Dash cayenne pepper, to taste
Pinch red pepper flakes

Instructions:

1. Combine vegetables in a quart pan and barely cover with organic Chicken Bone Broth. Bring to a rolling boil and turn down the heat to a strong simmer.

2. When the vegetables are soft, add spices and blend in food processor until nearly smooth, and adjust seasonings to your preference.

3. Serve with a garnish of red pepper flakes in each bowl.

Tip: serve with Nearly Vegan Skillet Corn Bread.

Granny's Granola

Beth
Yield: 2 cups

Homemade granola is too easy and too yummy to pass by. I believe that once you see how easy it is to do it, you will never buy packaged granola again. Once you master the basics of granola making, get crazy with different ingredients in different combinations. A baggie full of granola is always a good thing to carry around with you for those times when you need an energy boost.

Ingredients:

1½ cups rolled oats, gluten-free
¼ cup crushed nuts (you choose the nut, or try a blend)
2 tablespoons sprouted flaxseed
2 tablespoons maguey sap
2 tablespoons coconut oil, melted
¼ cup sprouted teff kernels, toasted, popped

Instructions:

1. Preheat oven to 350°F.

2. In a medium bowl, toss together oats, nuts, and flaxseeds.

3. In a separate bowl, whisk melted oil and maguey sap together until blended.

4. Stir oil-maguey mixture into oats and combine until all dry ingredients are coated.

5. On a flat baking pan, pour out the raw granola and spread evenly.

6. Bake for 5 minutes or until roasted as you like it. Shake the pan from side to side every couple of minutes to keep any bits from burning on the bottom of the pan.

7. To pop teff kernels, add to small skillet over a medium-high to high heat. Stir frequently until popped. Teff will pop very quickly, so keep them moving and don't burn them. Remove from heat and allow teff to cool on small plate.

8. Remove granola from oven and transfer to a medium-size bowl until cooled. Add popped teff.

Variations: experiment with adding dried coconut flakes (watch carefully so coconut does not burn), raisins (again, watch so raisins do not burn), chopped dried fruit, and/or hazelnut oil.

Guacamole

Chef Eddie
Yield: 2 cups

Who doesn't love good guacamole? No friend of mine, that is for sure. Serve guacamole as a dip, with eggs, chicken, or on top of black beans. There are so many great uses for this delicious recipe. Make twice as much as you think you need because people will steal it right out from under your nose while you are cooking.

Ingredients:
2 avocados, pitted, peeled, and chopped
1 jalapeño, seeded and chopped fine
½ red onion, diced
½ bunch cilantro, chopped
1 tablespoon cumin, ground
1 tablespoon powdered chili pepper, ancho, habanero, or pasilla
Sea salt, to taste
Cayenne pepper, to taste
Lime juice, fresh squeezed, to taste

Instructions:
1. In a mixing bowl, combine all ingredients except lime juice. Mix with a fork to the consistency you like guacamole. Some like it chunky, some like it pureed. It's up to you.

2. Spread it out on a sheet pan. This will let you season it evenly. It will probably taste a little bland. Add lime juice until it livens up, adjust salt and pepper. Put it back into the mixing bowl, put plastic wrap on top of the guacamole (not the top of the bowl), and refrigerate for 30 minutes.

3. Take it out and taste it again. You may feel like it needs a little more cumin or a little more chili powder. Add it. I have often found it tastes great, but just seems to be a little flat. Lime juice is usually my answer. Have some handy to add at the end.

Jambalaya

Chef Eddie
Serves: 4–6

In South Louisiana the following recipe is merely a suggestion. Jambalaya can have any-thing, in any quantity. No two will be alike. Use whatever ingredients in whatever propor-tion you like, but this is a good template. It's often used as a simple dish for serving large numbers of people or a way to use up leftovers. The truth is it's just a great dish with a lot of flavor. I love it and my kids love it; I just don't tell them what's in it.

Ingredients:
1 pound medium shrimp, peeled, deveined, and chopped
6 ounces chicken, diced or pulled
2 tablespoons Creole Seasoning Mix
2 tablespoons extra-virgin olive oil
8 ounces turkey sausage, sliced
Sea salt, to taste
Black pepper, to taste
½ cup tomatoes, chopped
½ cup poblano pepper, chopped
¼ cup celery, chopped
4 scallions, sliced thin
¾ cup brown rice
3½ cups Chicken Stock
½ cup onion, chopped
2 tablespoons garlic, chopped
3 bay leaves
1 teaspoon Vegan Worcestershire Sauce
Cayenne pepper, to taste

Instructions:
1. In 2 separate bowls, lightly season chicken and shrimp with 1 tablespoon Creole Seasoning Mix and set aside.

2. In a heavy-bottomed pot with a lid, heat oil over medium heat. Add sliced sausage and cook, stirring, for 5 minutes. Add chicken and cook for 2 more minutes or long enough to get some color in it. Note: if using pulled chicken, add it in later with shrimp.

3. Add 1 tablespoon Creole Seasoning Mix, sea salt, and black pepper. Sauté spices for 1 minute, and then add tomatoes. Cook, stirring for a few minutes to let some of the liquid from the tomatoes evaporate. Add poblano peppers, celery, onions, garlic, and most of the scallions (reserve some to garnish the top of the dish). Cook, stirring, for 5 minutes. Get some nice color in those vegetables.

4. Stir in brown rice and mix well. Cook for 2–3 minutes. Add Chicken Stock, bay leaves, Worcestershire, and cayenne pepper, turning the heat up to high, and bring to a fast-bubbling simmer. Reduce heat to low to keep it simmering, cover the pot, and cook for 45 minutes.

5. Remove lid and check the rice. It should be al dente. If it is still too firm, cook longer. When rice is tender, add shrimp, stir in, and continue to cook, covered, for 5 minutes. Taste for seasoning, and adjust if needed.

6. Serve the jambalaya in bowls with scallions sprinkled on top.

Mushroom-Stuffed Chicken

Chef Jay Nichols
Serves: 6

Jay, the son of Lisa Nichols of *The Secret*, visited our (Beth and Ivan) home over the summer while Ivan was healing. He watched me (Beth) prepare Misner Plan meals during the time he was with us with great interest. A young chef-in-training at Le Cordon Bleu, he was very curious about how and why I used certain ingredients. As I explained every step of the way, I asked him if he would like to have a couple of recipes in our cookbook. He said, "Sure!" and voilà.

Ingredients:

3 boneless, skinless, hormone- and antibiotic-free chicken breasts
Plain goat's or sheep's milk yogurt, to cover chicken
¼ teaspoon sea salt
¼ teaspoon black pepper
½ white onion, minced
8 ounces organic baby bella mushrooms, minced
1 tablespoon grapeseed oil
1 lemon
6 tablespoons extra-virgin olive oil (or enough to cover the chicken)
Cooking string

Instructions:

1. Place chicken in a large bowl, cover with yogurt, and season with salt and pepper. Cover and place in refrigerator to marinate for at least 1 hour or, better yet, overnight.

2. In a medium-size saucepan, add 1 tablespoon grapeseed oil and sauté onion and mushrooms until onions are translucent and mushrooms have released most of their liquids. Drain and dry mixture and set aside.

3. Preheat oven to 350°F.

4. Remove chicken from marinade and place on sterilized cutting board. Lay a line of mushroom-onion mixture lengthwise on each marinated chicken breast. Roll chicken with the sautéed mushroom and onion into "taquito" rolls, end over end. Secure with cooking string, making sure to leave no escape for the sautéed mixture inside.

5. Heat 3 tablespoons extra-virgin olive oil until shimmering in a heavy-bottomed pan. Pan cook chicken to brown outside, sealing in juices, and giving the chicken a nice golden brown color. Turn often to avoid overbrowning chicken pieces.

6. Place chicken rolls in oven and cook to internal temperature of 165°F. Check with meat thermometer.

7. Remove from oven and let rest for 10 minutes for liquids to settle.

8. To serve, remove string and cut across the grain at a slant for presentation.

Pico de Gallo

Chef Eddie
Serves: 4

Another way of making ordinary dishes pop is to serve with this Pico de Gallo. It goes well on top of fish or chicken, and even in salads.

Ingredients:

¾ pound tomatoes (about 2 medium or 1½ cups), seeded and finely diced
⅓ cup cilantro, chopped
¼ cup red onion, finely chopped
1 fresh jalapeño or serrano chili, finely chopped, including seeds for more taste
1 tablespoon lime juice, freshly squeezed (or more to taste)
2 teaspoons fine sea salt or 1 teaspoon kosher salt

Instructions:

1. Mix all ingredients together in a bowl and taste. Adjust seasoning as needed.

2. Place covered in the refrigerator for 1 hour. Taste, adjust seasonings, and serve.

Tip: When tasting, you are looking for a bright, crisp salsa. If it's flat, adding salt or lime juice will be your answer. To spice it up, you can add powdered chili, such as ancho or pasilla.

Poblano Sauce

Chef Eddie
Yield: 3 cups

It is always a good idea to make extra of this sauce and reserve for many other uses. Poblano is an underused vegetable. I particularly don't use green bell peppers a lot. I use poblanos. They seem to bring life to the party. This sauce will add life to many dishes, especially our Cashew Crusted Chicken Fingers.

Ingredients:
1 tablespoon extra-virgin olive oil
2 poblano peppers, roasted, peeled, seeded, and chopped
1 small onion, peeled, chopped, and caramelized
2 teaspoons minced garlic
1 teaspoon cumin
1 teaspoon powdered chili, such as ancho or pasilla
1 teaspoon sea salt
¼ teaspoon black pepper, freshly ground
3 cups Chicken Stock
3 tablespoons goat's or sheep's milk yogurt (optional)

Instructions:
1. Combine olive oil, roasted poblano, caramelized onion, and seasonings in medium sauce-pan over high heat and cook, stirring occasionally, for about 2 minutes.

2. Stir in Chicken Stock, bring to a boil, and cook over high heat for 10 minutes. Reduce heat to medium.

3. Stir in yogurt and simmer for 2 minutes.

4. Remove from heat and puree in a food processor or blender.

Tip: this can be made a day ahead and reheated.

To roast a poblano, place it on the burner of a gas stove until the skin blisters. When the skin is blistered all over, remove from the heat to a pot and put the top on. Let it rest for 15 minutes, and the skins will be falling off.

If you don't have a gas stove, use the broiler in your oven.

To serve: Place Cashew Crusted Chicken Fingers on a plate and spoon some sauce on the top. This can be done on individual plates or on a large serving platter.

Red Beans and Rice

Chef Eddie
Yield: 3 quarts

Talk about a New Orleans tradition. On any Monday, you can count on this being the special in many restaurants around town or on the dinner tables that night all across the city.

Ingredients:
1 poblano pepper
1 large yellow onion
2 stalks celery
1 yellow pepper
8 links spicy andouille chicken sausage (Applegate brand)
3–4 bay leaves
2 teaspoons sea salt
1 tablespoon Creole Seasoning Mix
1 pound red beans, soaked overnight
2 cloves garlic, minced
8 cups Chicken Stock
½ teaspoon cayenne pepper
1 sprig of fresh thyme
1 tablespoon fresh oregano, chopped
¼ teaspoon white pepper
Extra-virgin olive oil, for cooking

Instructions:
1. Dice all vegetables and the chicken sausage.

2. In a cast iron stockpot, cover the bottom with olive oil, then heat the pot for about 2 minutes over high heat. When the oil starts to shimmer, place all vegetables into the pot, with bay leaves, 1 teaspoon of the salt, 1 teaspoon of the Creole Seasoning Mix, and sauté until golden brown (about 7 minutes), scraping the bottom of the pot periodically.

3. Add red beans and garlic to the pot and continue to sauté for another 3 minutes, occasionally scraping the bottom of the pot.

4. Add Chicken Stock and remaining ingredients and bring to a simmer. Allow ingredients to simmer for about 1 hour. During the time it is simmering, give the beans a taste and adjust the seasoning, if desired. The level of the stock should stay about even with the top of or a little underneath the beans until they are done.

5. When done, the beans should be creamy in texture, spiced, and delicious. If they are still firm, then keep the stock level up and simmer a bit longer until the desired texture is reached.

6. For extra creaminess, I like to take an immersion blender and pulse it a few times in the pot of finished beans. Just be sure to remove the bay leaves and the thyme sprig before blending.

Tip: Ladle the beans over ½ cup cooked brown rice per person and top with a grilled chicken breast. Now that's comfort food.

Red Onion Rings

Chef Eddie
Yield: 1 cup

This pairs well with any kind of chicken or served with a baked sweet potato. Adding the crunchy rings to something soft will set your dish apart from the rest of the pack.

Ingredients:
1 cup red onion, peeled, cut in half, and pulled into rings
¼ cup yogurt, goat's or sheep's milk, for marinating
Grapeseed oil, for cooking
Creole Seasoning Mix, to taste

Instructions:
1. Marinate the onion rings in the yogurt for 15 minutes in the refrigerator. Onion rings should be really cold prior to going into the skillet.

2. Preheat heavy-bottomed, deep skillet to a medium-high heat. Add grapeseed oil and bring to temperature.

3. Pull the layers apart. Place in skillet for approximately 2–3 minutes. Look for a golden brown color. Do not allow to burn.

4. Pour out on a paper towel and spread them into a single layer.

5. Immediately sprinkle a little Creole Seasoning Mix on each piece and let them continue to crisp.

Tip: crisping time will depend on the humidity in your area.

Roasted Eggplant with Southwest Yogurt

Chef Eddie
Serves: 4

Eggplant can be tough for some people to enjoy. I've heard that Ivan and Beth are two of those people. Well, once you've tried this dish, you may change your tune. Roasting the eggplants brings out a depth of flavors, and saucing with the flavor-forward yogurt will add an extra bonus for your enjoyment. Prepare to be surprised.

Ingredients:
2 medium-size purple eggplants
Olive oil for brushing
½ cup Greek yogurt
½ bunch cilantro, chopped
2 teaspoon extra-virgin olive oil
1–2 cloves garlic, finely minced
Santa Fe seasoning, to taste
Sea salt and freshly cracked black pepper, to taste

Instructions:
1. Preheat oven to 350°F.

2. Slice eggplants lengthways. Score the cut side of the eggplants in a diagonal crisscross pattern, being careful not to cut the skin.

3. Place the eggplant slices on a baking tray and brush the cut and scored sides with olive oil.

4. Sprinkle with Santa Fe seasoning.

5. Place eggplants in the oven and roast for 30–45 minutes or until completely soft and nicely browned.

6. While eggplants are in the oven, mix together yogurt, extra-virgin olive oil, cilantro, garlic, Santa Fe seasoning. Taste and adjust seasoning until you are satisfied. Keep in the fridge until ready to use.

7. Once eggplants are completely roasted, remove to a plate. Dress with yogurt sauce or serve sauce on the side.

Roasted Red Peppers

Chef Eddie
Yield: 3–4 cups

Roasted red bell peppers can be a magic flavor enhancer to many dishes. The smokiness, sweetness, and slight pungency add another depth of flavor that is both unexpected and exciting.

Ingredients:

4 red peppers
Extra-virgin olive oil, for cooking

Instructions:

1. You can either char peppers on high heat on a gas range by placing them directly onto the grates, or roast them in the oven. Use tongs to turn peppers. Blacken on all sides whether you are cooking in the oven or on top of the stove.

2. If roasting in the oven, preheat oven broiler to 375°F. Arrange peppers on a cookie sheet and put them into the oven, turning every time the side facing the broiler is charred. Once done, place the peppers in a covered bowl, a brown paper bag, or a pot with a lid. As steam from the peppers condenses, the skin becomes easier to peel off.

3. Once peppers have cooled, carefully peel off blackened skin and discard. Pull or cut off the top of the pepper. Tear open pepper and remove seeds.

4. Resist rinsing or washing peppers, as water will diminish the flavor and remove some of the natural oils. When skins and seeds have been removed, they are ready to be used in your dish.

Tip: cover anything leftover in oil, adding garlic slices or herbs if desired, and refrigerate for up to 2 weeks.

Salmon Cobb Salad

Chef Eddie
Serves: 2

Another hearty, healthy salad that is a take on the traditional Cobb salad. Instead of the bacon, we are using salmon.

Ingredients:

3 ounces fresh salmon, chopped into chunks
Creole Seasoning Mix or Santa Fe Seasoning Mix
Extra-virgin olive oil, for cooking
2 boiled eggs, quartered
2 ounces roasted pepper, diced
2 ounces Parmesan cheese, diced
2 cups mixed greens
Sea salt, to taste
Black pepper, to taste

Instructions:

1. Sprinkle salmon with salt and pepper and then sprinkle a second time with either Creole or Santa Fe Seasoning Mix. Cut into large chunks.

2. Preheat a cast-iron skillet with enough oil to cover the bottom until oil in the pan just begins to shimmer.

3. Add salmon and cook until there is a nice color on the fish, about 2 minutes. Rotate salmon around until there is color on all sides, about another 2 minutes. Be careful not to overcook salmon; you are looking for medium doneness. When salmon is done, remove from the pan and allow to cool.

4. Toss greens with a little sea salt, pepper, and your favorite Misner Plan dressing and pour into the bottom of the salad serving bowl. Add straight, equal lines of eggs, salmon, peppers, and cheese and serve.

Salmon Tartare

Chef Eddie
Serves: 4–6

I love this for entertaining. It looks and sounds really high end, and the flavor backs it up. It's also a great treat that's really good for you to have for lunch or a light dinner. Fresh salmon has the richness and flavor to be decadent. Yet it's reasonably priced and doesn't take large quantities to feed many. There are two recipes here—one a little spicy and the other traditional and elegant. Why torture yourself deciding? Make both.

Spicy Salmon Tartare

Ingredients:
1 eight-ounce salmon filet, very fresh, diced
1 bunch cilantro, chopped fine, about 1 cup
½ red onion, minced
1 tablespoon organic Dijon mustard, such as Annie's brand with apple cider vinegar
1 tablespoon lime juice, freshly squeezed
1 tablespoon chipotle puree*
Sea salt, to taste
Black pepper, freshly ground, to taste

Traditional Salmon Tartare

Ingredients:
1 eight-ounce salmon filet, skinless
¼ cup cucumber, seeded, finely diced
1 tablespoon lime juice, freshly juiced
1½ teaspoons fresh chives, minced
1½ teaspoons fresh parsley or cilantro, minced
1½ teaspoons tea seed oil or grapeseed oil

1½ teaspoons jalapeño, seeded and minced
1½ teaspoons shallot, minced
¾ teaspoon fresh ginger, peeled and minced
¼ scant teaspoon lime zest
Sea salt, to taste
Cayenne or black pepper, freshly ground, to taste

Instructions:

1. Thinly cut salmon into ⅛-inch-wide dice.

2. Place salmon in a medium-size bowl and toss to incorporate all the other ingredients.

3. Season tartare to taste with sea salt and pepper and refrigerate for 30 minutes.

4. Taste again, adjust seasoning, and serve on very cold plates

*Note: to make an organic, vinegar- and sugar-free chipotle puree, rehydrate dried, organic chipotle peppers in filtered water and puree in the food processor.

Shrimp Creole

Chef Eddie
Serves: 8

This is South Louisiana's version of spaghetti and meatballs. It is also a great dish no matter where you're from. I served it as a sauce over fish to First Lady Michelle Obama and her guests aboard *Air Force 2* when they visited New Orleans.

Ingredients:

4 ounces ghee
2 cups onions, chopped
1 cup poblano peppers, chopped
1 cup celery, chopped
Sea salt, to taste
Cayenne pepper, to taste
2 bay leaves
4 cups fresh, ripe tomatoes, peeled, seeded, and chopped
1 tablespoon garlic, chopped
A few dashes Bragg's Liquid Aminos
2 tablespoons gluten-free flour blend
1 cup water
2½ pounds large shrimp, tail off, peeled, and deveined
½ cup scallions, chopped
2 tablespoons parsley, chopped
4 cups sprouted brown rice, cooked

Instructions:

1. Melt ghee in a large saucepan over medium heat.

2. Add onions, peppers, and celery to the pan. Let them start cooking up and then season the vegetables with sea salt and cayenne to taste. Start with ½ teaspoon sea salt and ⅛

teaspoon cayenne and go from there. What you are doing is layering your seasonings, rather than adding them all at the end. Sauté vegetables until they are wilted, about 6–8 minutes.

3. Stir in bay leaves, tomatoes, and garlic. Season with sea salt and cayenne. Start with ½ teaspoon sea salt and ⅛ teaspoon of cayenne. Taste as you go along to create the flavor you want. Bring mixture up to a boil and then reduce to a simmer. Simmer the mixture for about 15 minutes. If the mixture becomes too dry, add some water.

4. Whisk flour and water together. Add flour-water mixture to the tomato mixture and continue to cook for 4–6 minutes. Taste again and adjust your spices for the final time.

5. Serve as a stand-alone dish topped with chopped scallions and parsley and served over ¼ cup of sprouted brown rice, or as a great sauce for fish.

Shrimp Étouffée

Chef Jay Nichols
Serves: 4

Here is Chef Jay's second guest appearance. We think you will agree with us that he has a promising career ahead of him.

Ingredients:

4 tomatoes, diced
½ white onion, minced
1 shallot, minced
Black pepper, to taste
1 clove garlic, fresh minced
2 tablespoons grapeseed oil
Sea salt, to taste
2 pounds uncooked shrimp, peeled and deveined

Instructions:

1. To make tomato-based sauce, combine tomatoes, onion, shallot, black pepper, and garlic in a saucepan with 1 tablespoon grapeseed oil. Cook on low for 45 minutes until well blended and soft. Stir in sea salt to taste. Start with 1 teaspoon and increase amount, if needed. Strain into a medium-size bowl and set sauce aside.

2. Cook shrimp in a medium-size pan on low heat in 1 tablespoon grapeseed oil.

3. Finish by pouring tomato sauce over shrimp and simmering about 5 minutes. Serve with personal preference of Misner Plan garnish.

Southwest Baked Egg Muffins

Chef Eddie
Yield: 3 dozen

When prepared in advance, this grab-and-go recipe will come in handy when you don't have time to spend a lot of time in the morning getting breakfast ready. You may find that you even create reasons to claim to be in a hurry more often.

Ingredients:

½ cup shitake and portobello mushrooms, chopped (1 tablespoon per muffin)
¼ cup yellow peppers, diced (½ tablespoon per muffin)
¼ cup yellow onion, diced (½ tablespoon per muffin)
¼ teaspoon fine sea salt
⅛ teaspoon cayenne pepper
6 strips uncured turkey bacon
7 eggs
3 ounces sparkling water (or orange juice)
⅓ cup goat cheddar cheese, shredded (¾ tablespoon per muffin)
Ghee, as needed for cooking
Extra-virgin olive oil, as needed for cooking

Instructions:

1. Clean portobello mushrooms by removing stems and scraping all gills off the undersides. Remove stems of shitake mushrooms and then chop.

2. Spread olive oil on bottoms of muffin pan cups to prevent sticking (option, line with unbleached paper cups to help your muffins go portable).

3. Sauté yellow peppers and onions in cast-iron skillet on medium-high heat. Add salt and cayenne pepper. After they are translucent and wilted, remove to a separate dish and put mushrooms in a skillet and sauté. If skillet gets too dry, add ghee.

4. Heat cast-iron skillet to high. Reduce heat to medium high and lay 5 pieces of turkey bacon in the bottom. Bacon should sizzle. If the bacon starts to spit, reduce heat a little more. After about 2 minutes, flip the bacon. When it looks crispy, take bacon off heat and line the inside of each cup of muffin pan with the bacon.

5. Whisk eggs together with sparkling water or orange juice.

6. Use a 3-ounce ladle to add scrambled egg mixture to each muffin cup. Add ½ tablespoon yellow peppers, ½ tablespoon yellow onion, and 1 tablespoon shitake and portobello mushrooms to each cup. Add ¾ tablespoon goat cheese on top.

7. Bake in the oven for 16 minutes.

8. Remove and serve for a tasty breakfast.

Southwest Pasta Salad

Chef Eddie
Serves: 2

This variation on the pasta makes for a great lunch or dinner. It is vegetarian as prepared here, but don't be afraid to add grilled shrimp or chicken.

Basic "Pasta"

Ingredients:
1 jalapeño or poblano pepper, seeded, stemmed, and minced
1 Haas avocado, pitted, removed from skin, and diced
1 tablespoon powdered chili pepper, ancho, habanero, or anaheim
1 tablespoon cumin
½ teaspoon sea salt
½ bunch cilantro, chopped
Lime juice, freshly squeezed from ½ lime
1 medium-size heirloom tomato, seeded and diced
3 tablespoons non-GMO corn kernels, blanched
Extra-virgin olive oil, cilantro oil, or Portuguese Hot Sauce, to finish

Instructions:
1. Make Basic "Pasta" and spread on a baking sheet to cool. (Spreading on a baking sheet will allow even distribution of other ingredients.)

2. Spread the rest of the ingredients over pasta on a baking sheet until you get the ratios you like. The jalapeños, avocado, tomatoes, cilantro, and corn should all be scattered in quantities so that you will get some in every bite. Add or subtract as you feel necessary. If you like things less spicy, back off the jalapeño or use poblano instead.

3. Adjust seasonings and squeeze in lime juice.

4. Drizzle with oil or Portuguese Hot Sauce to finish.

Spinach Avocado Soup (Cold)

Chef Eddie
Serves: 2

This raw soup is packed with antioxidants and tons of flavor. What an easy way to eat your vegetables. When I say easy, I mean the preparation of this soup is *really* easy.

Ingredients:
2 cups packed spinach leaves
1 avocado, pitted and removed from peel
1 medium cucumber, cubed
2 large cloves garlic
½-inch piece fresh ginger, peeled
Pinch sea salt
Pinch cayenne pepper
2 tablespoons lemon juice, freshly squeezed
1 cup water
Sprouts, for serving (optional)

Instructions:
1. Place all ingredients in a blender on high until smooth.

2. If soup is too thick, thin with water.

3. Pour into serving bowls. Top with sprouts to garnish.

Sweet Potato Cakes with Santa Fe Crema

Chef Eddie
Yield: 6 ½-cup patties

The mushrooms add a texture to these bean cakes that creates a burger of sorts. Serve as a stand-alone dish or on top of a green salad, topped with the crema, as a deconstructed sandwich.

Ingredients:
1 large or 2 medium sweet potatoes
3½ tablespoons extra-virgin olive oil
⅛ cup oyster mushrooms, coarsely chopped
⅛ cup shitake mushrooms, coarsely chopped
1 teaspoon sea salt (keep ⅛ teaspoon separate for seasoning the mushrooms)
⅛ teaspoon cayenne pepper
1½ cups cooked quinoa
1 teaspoon cumin
1 teaspoon chili powder
½ red onion, minced
1 tablespoon chipotle puree (jarred, not canned)
1 egg, beaten
¼ cup gluten-free panko
1 tablespoon coconut or olive oil for baking
6 tablespoons Santa Fe Crema

Instructions:
1. Preheat oven to 350°F.

2. On an oven pan, roast the sweet potatoes until done, about 45 minutes. The potatoes should still have a touch of firmness, if possible. Remove from the oven and allow the potatoes to cool.

3. When the potatoes are cool, the skins should peel right off, leaving the flesh of the potato. Mash sweet potato flesh until very few lumps are left, but take care not to overdo it. Too much handling will make them nearly liquefy. We're making patties, not soup.

4. Heat the skillet to high heat with 2–3 tablespoons olive oil until the oil begins to shimmer.

5. Reduce heat to medium high. Add the mushrooms and sauté until soft, about 12 minutes. Season with salt and a little cayenne, then set aside. Feel free to add a little cumin and chili powder if you like. The mushrooms should be very flavorful. If you are using button, cremini, or portobello mushrooms, they will release their water. Keep the mushrooms in the pan long enough to reduce or cook that liquid away. Also, if you're using a cast-iron skillet, you may also have to add a little olive oil to the pan as you're cooking if it gets too dry.

6. In a large bowl, mix mashed sweet potato, quinoa, cumin, chili powder, salt, cayenne pepper, red onion, and chipotle puree until well incorporated. Cover and set aside in the fridge for 15 minutes to allow the mixture to develop its flavor.

7. Remove the mixture from refrigerator. Form the mixture into 6 patties.

8. Dip the patties in beaten egg, then coat with gluten-free panko.

9. Spray the breaded patties with coconut or olive oil and place them directly on your oven's baking rack over an oven pan.

10. Bake for about 15 minutes or until breading is nicely browned and crunchy.

11. Remove from the pan and serve immediately topped with 1 tablespoon of Santa Fe Crema on each patty.

Sweet Potato Hash Browns

Chef Eddie
Serves: 4–6

A good breakfast deserves good hash browns. As an extra bonus, these are Misner Plan approved.

Ingredients:

3 poblano peppers, roasted and peeled, seeded and stemmed
2 tablespoons extra-virgin olive oil
1 small red onion, thinly sliced
2 tablespoons ghee
2 medium sweet potatoes, peeled and cut into ¼-inch dice or grated
3 garlic cloves, thinly sliced
1 rosemary sprig
2 tablespoons lemon juice, freshly squeezed
Sea salt, to taste
Black pepper, freshly ground, to taste

Instructions:

1. Roast poblano peppers directly over a gas flame or under a preheated broiler, turning, until charred all over. Transfer to bowl, cover tightly with plastic wrap, and let cool. Peel, seed, and stem poblanos and then thinly slice them.

2. In large skillet, heat olive oil. Add onion and cook, stirring, until golden, about 5 minutes.

3. Add ghee, sweet potatoes, garlic, and rosemary and cook over moderate heat, stirring occasionally until the potatoes are tender and lightly browned, about 10 minutes.

4. Stir in poblanos and lemon juice, season with salt and pepper. Discard rosemary sprig and serve.

Tip: top hash browns with a poached egg for each person, and you have a fantastic brunch.

Thai Cashew Slaw

Chef Eddie
Yield: 1 pint

Thai food has always been interesting to me—lots of fresh flavors going on at the same time, crisp ingredients, all with a good amount of heat. It definitely makes your mouth happy! This slaw has everything going for it. Texture, lots of flavor, some heat, and it's good for you. What else could you want?

You can eat the slaw by itself, use it on fish tacos, serve it with scallops, chicken, duck—well you get my drift. In this dish we use it together with a jazzed up quinoa to make a great compliment of grains and vegetables.

I am also pretty sure you will want to keep a supply of the Thai Cashew Butter Sauce on hand just because.

Ingredients:
1½ cups red cabbage, shredded
1 red bell pepper, diced
½ red onion, diced
1 cup carrots, shredded
½ cup cilantro, chopped
¼ cup scallions, diced
½ cup cashew halves
½ teaspoon fine sea salt
1 teaspoon extra-virgin olive oil
1 teaspoon fresh lime juice
3 tablespoons mint
¼ cup Thai Cashew Butter Sauce

Instructions:

1. Combine all ingredients except Thai Cashew Butter Sauce and cashews in large mixing bowl to create slaw.

2. Just before serving, add Thai Cashew Butter Sauce and cashews and toss to combine.

3. Give it a taste and adjust seasonings.

Variation: you can create this dish using quinoa in place of shredded cabbage for a Thai Quinoa Pilaf.

Turkey Chili

Beth
Serves: 10

After finishing Phases 1 and 2, Ivan and I were hungry for a hearty, spicy chili. Before Ivan's diagnosis, I was used to opening canned chili or picking up a seasoning packet at the store to add to the basic ingredients. No more. This recipe is hearty, filling, and great to prepare when expecting company. (Please note, to my fellow Texans, I know this chili has beans. You'll have to forgive my indiscretion with this one.)

Ingredients:
5 cups red beans
¾ cup water
4 large tomatoes, chopped
2 teaspoons sea salt
1 pound ground turkey
1 tablespoon extra-virgin olive oil
½ onion, diced
3 cloves garlic, minced
1 teaspoon cayenne
2 teaspoons cumin

Instructions:
1. Sort and rinse red beans. Place in a large bowl (beans will swell) and cover with water. Cover with plastic wrap. Check beans often as they soak and add water as needed. Soak for about 8 hours and then drain, rinse, and cook on low heat, keeping beans on a low, rolling boil, until tender, about 40 minutes. Drain off cooking water and reserve beans to one side.

2. In 2-quart pan, add water, tomatoes, and ½ teaspoon of the sea salt. Boil tomatoes about 10 minutes on a low, rolling boil. Process tomatoes until smooth in a food processor. Reserve to one side.

3. Brown ground turkey on low heat until cooked through, stirring frequently. Add beans and tomato sauce and allow them to simmer.

4. Cook onion and garlic on low heat in olive oil until translucent.

5. Add onion and garlic to the meat mixture and season with spices and the remainder of sea salt. Cook on low heat for about 20 minutes. Taste and adjust the spices according to your taste.

Veggie Meatballs

Chef Eddie
Serves: 4–6

This recipe is quite versatile. You can serve this as traditional meatballs and spaghetti using einkorn pasta or veggie pasta and a great fresh tomato sauce like Sauce Piquant. You can use the meatballs chopped up as taco filling, just season them with cumin and chili powder. If the mixture were pressed into a patty, it would make a great veggie burger or sausage patty, depending how you season it.

The first step is to prepare the veggies to make the "meatballs."

Ingredients:

3 cups portobello, shitake, and trumpet mushrooms (or whatever you like), finely chopped. Shitake and trumpets will be firmer for better texture. Include the stems.
1 medium (3 cups) purple eggplant, peeled and roughly chopped
2 medium (3 cups) yellow onion, cut into large chunks
¼ cup extra-virgin olive oil
2 tablespoons balsamic vinegar
2 teaspoons chopped garlic
Sea salt, to taste

Instructions:

1. Preheat oven to 350°F.

2. Add chopped mushrooms, stems and all, to your food processor and pulse three times or until finely chopped, about the size of a black bean. Don't overload the food processor. If you have a smaller machine, do this in batches. Overloaded bowls will make the vegetables on the bottom very fine, and the top will still be chunky.

3. Place processed mushrooms onto large, parchment-lined, 17- x 12-inch rimmed baking sheet. Pulse roughly chopped eggplant in food processor in the same manner. Place eggplant onto sheet pan with mushrooms.

4. Repeat this process with onion. Mound mushrooms, eggplant, and onions together.

5. Drizzle the mound of mushrooms, eggplant, and onion with the olive oil and vinegar. Using your hands, toss it all together. Spread the mixture evenly over the sheet pan. Sprinkle in the chopped garlic powder and pepper. Add sea salt to taste.

6. Bake for a total of 20 minutes, remove the mixture from the oven, and let it cool. (Keep the oven on.)

The second step is to complete the dish.

Ingredients:

1 cup shredded Parmesan or Pecorino cheese
½ cup gluten-free bread crumbs, or panko
2 cups veggie "meatball" mixture
2 large eggs, beaten
½ cup coconut milk or Cashew Cream, savory variation
½ teaspoon red pepper flakes
½ teaspoon ground white pepper
½ teaspoon fresh oregano, minced
1 tablespoon fresh parsley, minced
½ teaspoon sea salt
Olive oil for baking

Instructions:

1. In a large bowl, combine cheese, bread crumbs, veggie "meatball" mixture, eggs, coconut milk, red pepper flakes, white pepper, oregano, parsley, and salt. Allow mixture to stand for 30 minutes.

2. On parchment-lined, 17- x 12-inch rimmed baking sheet, make a whole bunch of little meatballs. Drizzle or spray meatballs with olive oil. Place pan in the still-hot oven.

3. After 15 minutes, check meatballs for firmness. Continue cooking until firm, maybe 5 more minutes.

Zucchini Fries

Chef Eddie
Yield: 3 cups

Most zucchini fries are not Misner Plan friendly, so having this recipe will make you smile. These fries won't crush you on the calories; just don't cut the zucchini too thin.

Ingredients:
3 cups zucchini, sliced into pencil-thick fries or thicker
1 teaspoon sea salt
1 teaspoon Italian seasoning
½ cup garbanzo bean flour
1 egg, beaten
¼ cup almond milk
1½ cups gluten-free bread crumbs or gluten-free panko
¼ cup extra-virgin olive oil

Instructions:
1. Preheat oven to 415°F.

2. In a large bowl, sprinkle the zucchini fries with salt and Italian seasoning or the seasoning of your choice. Or try Santa Fe Seasoning Mix or Creole Seasoning Mix; you'll love it.

3. Add garbanzo bean flour and toss to coat.

4. Set up two bowls, one with egg and almond milk whisked together, and the other with panko.

5. Dip each zucchini stick into egg-and-milk mixture, and then roll it in gluten-free bread crumbs or gluten-free panko.

6. Place in single layer on a parchment-lined baking sheet until you've used all zucchini. Drizzle or spray coated fries with olive oil.

7. Bake for 20 minutes.

8. Garnish and serve.

Zucchini Fritters

Chef Eddie
Yield: 8

Similar to a rösti, a combination of zucchini and buckwheat make these a delicious, savory appetizer.

Ingredients:
2–3 whole zucchini, shredded, 4 cups total
¼ cup red onion, shredded
1 egg
¼ cup buckwheat flour
¼ teaspoon Homemade Baking Soda
¼ teaspoon garlic powder
¼ cup grated Parmesan cheese
Sea salt, to taste
Black pepper, freshly cracked, to taste
Grapeseed oil, for cooking

Instructions:
1. Place grated zucchini and red onion on a thin dishtowel. Wring out all the water until you have a very dry mixture.

2. Combine zucchini and red onion with the remaining ingredients (except oil for cooking) and toss until all the ingredients are incorporated.

3. Heat oil in a cast-iron skillet until hot.

4. Using a spoon, scoop small piles of mixture into the oil. Cook quickly on each side until golden brown.

5. Remove to a cooling rack lined with paper towels.

6. Serve immediately with your favorite Misner Plan sauce or dressing.

Twenty-Nine

Beth's Healing Body Bars

Beth
Yield: 12

We love to take these bars with us on our travels or to networking mixers. When what is being served is not on the Misner Plan, we won't go hungry with these filling Healing Body Bars.

Ingredients:

2 cups gluten-free oats
2 tablespoons sprouted flax meal, freshly ground
½ cup gluten-free flour blend
1 teaspoon cinnamon
⅛ teaspoon sea salt
⅓ cup raw pistachios, shelled and chopped
⅓ cup mixed raw sprouted nuts, crushed
1½ ounces raisins
⅔ cup raw, sprouted almond butter

¼ cup maguey sap
¼ cup pureed dates
⅛ cup grapeseed oil

Instructions

1. Preheat oven to 450°F.

2. Toast gluten-free oats on a natural stone sheet pan for about 5 minutes or until lightly browned. If using a metal sheet pan, check sooner for browning. Shake sheet pan every 2 minutes to avoid burning oats. Remove from oven and allow to cool slightly while mixing dry ingredients together. Adding toasted oats while warm will soften almond butter and make it easier to combine your ingredients more thoroughly.

3. Turn the oven down to 350°F.

4. In a large bowl, mix flax meal with flour, cinnamon, and sea salt. Stir in pistachios, mixed nuts, and raisins, and mix dry ingredients together well.

5. Puree dates by simmering 5 large pitted dates in a small amount of water, then puree with an emulsion immersion blender. In a medium-size bowl, whisk together maguey sap, pureed dates, and grapeseed oil. Incorporate almond butter into mixture and add warm, toasted oats. Stir until incorporated well.

6. Pour into dry ingredients and mix until ingredients begin to stick together.

7. Turn batter onto the natural stone sheet pan you toasted the oats on and press smooth. Mixture should be about ½-inch thick. Bake for 12–15 minutes or until lightly browned.

8. Remove from oven and cut into bars with a pizza cutter while still warm. Cut carefully, so as not to scratch the baking stone. Loosen from the pan and allow bars to cool completely before wrapping in wax paper.

Tip: Bars may be kept on the counter if you plan to consume them quickly. Otherwise, put bars into ziplock bags and keep in the fridge for about 2 weeks.

*Notes: you can vary the type of nuts you use and add other spices, such as nutmeg, pumpkin pie spice, and/or cloves. You may omit raisins or use chopped dried figs, sulfur-free dried apricots, or other chopped dried fruits according to your tastes. I don't recommend dried cranberries, as it is nearly impossible to find them without sugar added or even Red #40. You may wish to add unsweetened coconut flakes. And honey may be substituted for one of the sweeteners, if you prefer.

There is a lot of room for variety with this recipe. Just be sure your batter holds together somewhat before pressing it onto the cookie sheet, or you will end up with a tasty granola, but you won't have energy bars.

BORA (Banana-Oatmeal-Raisin-Almond) Cookies

Beth
Yield: 1 dozen

These cookies surprised me the first time I made them. They turned out so airy and light with a shiny, smooth surface. They have quickly become our favorite grab-and-go quick snack for those times when we need to stretch the amount of time between lunch and supper.

Ingredients:

1 cup creamy almond butter
¼ cup maguey sap
⅛ cup coconut oil
1 large egg, beaten
1 ripe banana, mashed
1 teaspoon ground cinnamon
¾ teaspoon baking soda
½ teaspoon sea salt
1½ cup gluten-free rolled oats
2 tablespoons gluten-free flour blend
½ cup raisins

Instructions:

1. Preheat oven to 350°F.

2. In a medium-size bowl, mix together almond butter, maguey sap, coconut oil, egg, and banana.

3. In a small bowl, stir together ground cinnamon, baking soda, sea salt, rolled oats, and flour.

4. Gently add dry ingredients to the wet ingredients, stirring until combined, and then fold in raisins. Give the mixture a quick stir to distribute fruit well.

5. Drop the mixture onto a cookie sheet by the spoonful and press into flat rounds with the back of a fork.

6. Bake for 12–14 minutes or until lightly browned. Allow it to cool for 10 minutes before transferring them to a plate and serving them to your eagerly awaiting friends and family.

Variation: stir in ¼ cup of chopped walnuts with raisins before spooning onto cookie sheet.

Chewy Spiced Ginger Bites

Beth
Yield: 12

I wanted something to cook to have with Chef Eddie's Sea Salt Caramel Yogurt and thought of a type of ginger cookie. This recipe resulted from what ingredients I had on hand, and their chewy softness and delightful ginger flavor was just perfect. Don't expect a crisp ginger snap when you make these.

Ingredients:

1 cup raw, sprouted almond butter
3 tablespoons raw coconut nectar
2 large eggs, room temperature
2 teaspoons ginger root, freshly grated
¾ cup coconut sugar
¼ cup coconut flour
1 teaspoon baking soda
½ teaspoon ground ginger
¾ teaspoon cinnamon
¼ teaspoon ground allspice
½ teaspoon sea salt
Pinch of black pepper, freshly ground

Instructions:

1. Preheat oven to 350°F.

2. Line two stoneware cookie pans with parchment paper.

3. Blend together almond butter, raw coconut nectar, eggs, and ginger until smooth.

4. In a medium-size bowl, sift together coconut sugar, coconut flour, baking soda, ginger, cinnamon, allspice, salt, and pepper.

5. Slowly add sugar and spice mixture to almond butter mixture while blending on low until just combined.

6. Drop the dough by rounded teaspoons about 2 inches apart on prepared baking sheets.

7. Bake cookies until firm around the edges and starting to crack in the center (cookies will look slightly puffed, but will flatten and crack more as they cool), about 8 minutes. Cool 2 minutes on the stoneware, then lift out parchment paper with cookies and transfer to wire racks to cool completely.

8. Serve with Sea Salt Caramel Yogurt or snack on them by themselves.

Chocolate Mousse

Beth
Serves: 6

This decadent and delightful mousse will please even the most discriminating chocolate lovers. And they won't believe what the secret ingredient is! Don't tell them until they have a chance to enjoy the rich, creamy chocolate goodness.

Ingredients:

2 large ripe, but not overly so, avocados
½ cup unsweetened cacao powder
½ cup maguey sap or coconut nectar
Dash of cinnamon
3 egg whites
½ pint of fresh raspberries

Instructions:

1. Blend avocados, cacao powder, maguey sap or coconut nectar, and cinnamon on medium-low speed until completely smooth.

2. Beat 3 egg whites until peaks form, then fold in to the chocolate mixture.

3. Spoon into small dessert cups and refrigerate until firm (about 3 hours).

4. Garnish with fresh raspberries and serve.

5. Sit back and watch the joy and delight on your guests' faces.

Flatbread

Beth
Yield: 8–10

When Ivan and I were nearing the end of our long Phase 2, we wanted to be able to eat some kind of a sandwich. So I experimented with some unleavened bread recipes until I was able to create just the right combination to make a flatbread that would substitute well for bread. The trick with this is not to eat too many slices at one sitting. Make up the recipe and then freeze half the batch to enjoy next week.

Ingredients:
2 cups gluten-free flour blend
1 teaspoon sea salt
¼ teaspoon garlic powder
¼ teaspoon Italian seasoning
⅓ cup grapeseed oil
⅔ cup water

Instructions:
1. Mix together flour and spices. To ⅓ cup grapeseed oil, add water to measure 1 cup and whisk together. Pour water and oil mixture into the flour and spice mixture and incorporate ingredients quickly with a slotted spoon or a fork.

2. Roll dough into balls about the size of walnuts and set aside. Place ⅓ cup baking-flour mix on a clean counter surface or cutting board. Taking dough balls one at a time, toss in the flour so you can flatten the balls between your palms into flat rounds, about ½-inch thick. Handle them carefully, as dough will stretch and tear easily.

3. Cook in lightly oiled cast-iron skillet or griddle over medium heat, turning when golden on one side. Remove from the pan when golden on the other side.

4. Enjoy hot, dipped in olive oil and sea salt, or allow to cool and use in place of sandwich bread.

Tip: This flatbread can be made with a variety of spices. Experiment with rosemary, basil, and roasted garlic bits to create the perfect savory bread, or omit garlic powder and Italian seasoning and add raisins and cinnamon for a breakfast treat.

Flourless Chocolate Zucchini Muffins

Beth
Serving size: 18

These rich, dark muffins are loaded with good nutrition and are not too sweet. They are best enjoyed fresh from the oven. Avoid the temptation to eat them every day once you make them. We like to freeze half the batch to enjoy later in the month.

Ingredients:

¼ cup plus 1 tablespoon coconut flour
1 tablespoon tapioca starch
½ cup almond flour
¼ cup organic cacao powder
1 teaspoon Homemade Baking Powder
¼ teaspoon sea salt
¼ cup coconut oil, warmed until liquid
4 large eggs at room temperature
¼ cup maguey sap
¼ cup coconut milk
½ teaspoon powdered vanilla
1 cup grated zucchini (1 small to medium zucchini)
3.5 ounces dark chocolate (70 percent or more cacao), chopped, divided in two parts

Instructions:

1. Preheat oven to 350°F. Line a muffin pan with paper cup liners.

2. In large bowl, sift together flours, cacao powder, Homemade Baking Powder, and sea salt.

3. In a smaller bowl, whisk together the coconut oil and eggs for a minute or so, until frothy.

4. Add the maguey sap, coconut milk, and powdered vanilla. Whisk to combine well.

5. Add wet ingredients to dry ingredients, and mix until well incorporated.

6. Squeeze the water out of grated zucchini and gently fold into the batter mixture along with half the chocolate chunks.

7. Spoon batter into prepared muffin cups, and sprinkle the tops evenly with the rest of the chocolate chunks.

8. Bake for 20-25 minutes, or until a toothpick comes out clean and the top springs back when pressed lightly.

9. Let cool for five to ten minutes in the pan, then lift muffins out gently and transfer to a rack to cool completely.

Flourless Nut Bread

Beth
Serving size: one loaf

Prior to Ivan's diagnosis, we had been on an African safari in South Africa. The chef at our camp, Camp Jabulani, made a delicious nut loaf that we both enjoyed greatly. Since we have reduced the amount of flour in our diet now, I have been able to recreate a version of the nut loaf with absolutely no traditional flours at all. Made with nut flour and ground nuts, this will be a crowd pleaser.

Ingredients:
1 ½ cups organic blanched almond flour
½ cup non-GMO organic corn starch
¼ cup organic flax meal
½ teaspoon sea salt
½ teaspoon baking soda
4 large eggs
2 teaspoons raw, organic agave nectar or honey
1 teaspoon Bragg's apple cider vinegar
¼ cup walnuts, coarsely chopped
¼ cup toasted almonds, coarsely chopped
¼ cup pistachios, coarsely chopped
¼ cup sunflower seeds
¼ cup black sesame seeds

Instructions:
1. Preheat oven to 350°F.

2. In a medium bowl, combine almond flour, corn starch, flax meal, salt and baking soda.

3. In a larger bowl, blend eggs 3-5 minutes until frothy. Stir in agave and vinegar.

4. Mix dry ingredients into wet, then add nuts and seeds and combine well.

5. Grease bottom of 7.5- x 3.5-inch loaf pan with coconut oil, and gently transfer the batter into the pan.

6. Bake for 30 minutes, or until a toothpick inserted into center of loaf comes out clean.

7. Cool and serve with ghee or our one of our dressings for dipping.

Key Lime Pie Bars

Beth
Yield: 20

I served these bars at a large public event and asked the participants to guess what the main ingredient was. They could not believe it when I revealed it was avocado. This is a nice treat to have on a rare occasion, and it is perfect to serve to guests or take to potlucks.

Crust

Ingredients:
1¼ cups macadamia nuts
1¼ cups pecans
¼ teaspoon vanilla
⅛ teaspoon sea salt
¼ cup well-packed, finely chopped dates

Instructions:
1. Grease 9-inch baking pan with raw, unscented coconut butter.

2. Process macadamia nuts, pecans, vanilla, and salt until small and crumbly in the food processor.

3. Continue processing while adding small amounts of chopped dates until crust sticks together.

4. Press crust into the greased baking dish.

Filling

Ingredients:
¾ cup fresh lime juice
7½ ounces avocado, ripe, but not overly so
½ cup plus 1 tablespoon coconut nectar
¼ cup plus 2 tablespoons coconut milk
½ teaspoon powdered vanilla
⅛ teaspoon fine sea salt
2 tablespoons liquid lecithin, non-GMO
½ cup plus 1 tablespoon raw, unscented coconut butter
½ cup Meringue
Mint leaves (garnish)

Instructions:
1. Blend all ingredients except lecithin and coconut butter until smooth. Add lecithin and coconut butter, blending until well incorporated.

2. Pour into the prepared crust and set it in the fridge/freezer (for about 1 hour) until firm.

3. Once set, spread a thin layer of Meringue on top.

4. Cut into bars and serve with a mint leaf garnish on each bar.

Meringue

Beth
Yield: 36 cookies

This honey-sweetened, sugar-free Meringue is just right for topping our Key Lime Pie Bars. Make cookies out of it for those times when you feel like you need a bit of a sweet treat.

Ingredients:
5 egg whites
¼ plus ⅛ teaspoon cream of tartar
1 tablespoon raw honey

Instructions:
1. Beat egg whites together with the cream of tartar to the point that the whites just begin to form soft peaks.

2. Slowly add honey while continuing to beat the mixture until stiff peaks form.

At this point, you have the Meringue you would use for topping our Key Lime Bars. To make Meringue Cookies, continue:

1. Preheat oven to 215°F.

2. Line two baking stones or cookie sheets with parchment paper.

3. Spoon drops of beaten egg whites onto prepared stones or cookie sheets.

4. Bake for about 2 hours or until cookies barely begin to brown.

5. Turn off oven and leave cookies in warm oven to brown to desired color.

Mexican Chocolate Torte

Beth
Serves: 8

This chocolate cake is good enough to take to a bake sale, if you can keep your family from devouring it as soon as it comes out of the oven. We like having it on a weekend morning with a cup of tea in place of a Starbucks muffin. A word of advice: you may wish to adjust the cayenne pepper to suit your taste buds.

Ingredients:
⅓ cup organic cacao powder
⅓ cup + 1 Tablespoon organic coconut flour
½ teaspoon sea salt
½ teaspoon organic baking soda
1 teaspoon organic ground cinnamon
½ teaspoon organic ground cayenne
6 pasture-raised, organic large eggs at room temperature
½ cup raw organic blue agave or organic coconut nectar
½ cup raw local honey
2 teaspoon organic vanilla extract
3 ounces unsweetened organic chocolate, melted
½ cup organic coconut oil

Instructions:
1. Preheat oven to 325°F.

2. Line 5- x 9-inch cake pan with parchment paper. Lightly oil paper with coconut oil.

3. Sift cacao, coconut flour, baking soda, sea salt, cinnamon, and cayenne into a small bowl.

4. Melt chocolate in a double boiler using a wooden spoon to stir often. Add coconut oil until it becomes liquid, stirring together with melted chocolate.

5. In a Vitamix, combine eggs, honey, molasses, and vanilla. Pulse a few times to mix together. Add melted chocolate and coconut oil mixture and blend on medium for 1 minute.

6. Add dry ingredients to the food processor and pulse to mix.

7. Turn batter gently into prepared cake pan and bake for 1 hour. Test with a toothpick after 45 minutes and watch carefully at the end of cooking, so the cake does not burn.

8. Let the cake cool completely in the pan. Remove from the pan by loosening the edges with a spatula and turning the cake out onto a flat serving tray. Carefully remove parchment paper. Cut into slices or squares.

Muffin Man Muffins

Beth
Yield: about 10

"Do you know the muffin man, the muffin man, the muffin man?" My mom used to sing this little ditty to us while making muffins when we were growing up. This song came to my mind when I was creating this delicious muffin recipe for Ivan so he could have muffins while he was healing.

Ingredients:

1 cup gluten-free rolled oats
1 cup unsweetened cherry juice
¼ cup maguey sap
¼ cup pureed banana
¼ cup coconut oil
¼ teaspoon sea salt
1 cup gluten-free flour blend
½ teaspoon cinnamon
3 teaspoons Homemade Baking Powder
½ cup raspberries

Instructions:

1. Preheat oven to 425°F.

2. Stir together oats and cherry juice and let stand while mixing wet ingredients.

3. Mix maguey, pureed banana, coconut oil, and salt until well incorporated.

4. Combine flour, cinnamon, and Baking Powder and add to oats/juice mixture. Fold in raspberries, and stir together gently until mixed.

5. Spoon the batter into a paper-lined stoneware muffin pan or muffin tin, and bake for 20–25 minutes, until a toothpick inserted in the middle of a muffin comes out dry.

Rhubarb Crumble

Beth

Serves: 4

This spin on Grandma's rhubarb pie is delicious enough to serve to even your most discerning guests. We enjoy this served warm or cold—whatever we are in the mood for.

Ingredients:

6 rhubarb stalks, chopped into 1-inch pieces
½ cup maguey sap
1 cup Granny's Granola

Instructions:

1. Preheat oven to 350°F.

2. In a small saucepan, pour maguey sap over rhubarb chunks. Simmer about 15 minutes, or until rhubarb begins to soften and fall apart.

3. Spoon mixture into dessert cups, pour 1 tablespoon warm maguey sap over each portion, and sprinkle with cinnamon.

4. Sprinkle tops with Granny's Granola and serve.

Variations: top with dollop of plain yogurt, goat's or sheep's milk; to make apple crumble, substitute chopped apples for the rhubarb and reduce the sap by half. Add cinnamon while simmering.

Rosemary Walnut Crackers

Beth
Yield: about 20

Who knew delicious, fresh crackers could be so easy to make and, oh, so good? Ivan and I love the contrast of sweet and savory with the herbs and raisins combined. I serve these crackers with Firecracker Soup.

Ingredients:

1 cup almond meal
½ tablespoon extra-virgin olive oil
2 tablespoons water
½ teaspoon sea salt
2 tablespoons raisins
12 walnut halves (split into one group of 8 and one group of 4)
1 sprig rosemary, remove leaves from the woody stem
Grapeseed oil for baking

Instructions:

1. Preheat oven to 350°F.

2. Pulse in food processor until combined thoroughly: almond meal, olive oil, water, sea salt, raisins, 8 walnut halves, rosemary.

3. When ingredients are combined, drop in 4 more walnuts and pulse until they are roughly chopped into the mixture. You will want to see larger chunks of nuts in the dough.

4. Scoop stiff dough out of the food processor bowl and form it into the shape of a large ball. Roll the dough out between 2 sheets of parchment paper until about ⅛-inch thick. Cut into squares with a pizza cutter. Take the end pieces and re-form them into a square so you can cut more crackers.

5. Lightly oil baking stone or cookie sheet with grapeseed oil. Spread the crackers out and cook about 15 minutes. Check them at 8 minutes and rotate the pan in the oven, if needed. They should brown lightly before you remove them from the oven.

6. Turn out on a wire rack to cool.

Scones

Beth
Serving size: 8-12 scones

This recipe makes such delicious Misner Plan scones that you'll need to pace yourself when eating them. The key is to share with others! We share tips below for adapting this recipe for savory scones that are just as delicious.

Ingredients:

2 ½ cups sprouted gluten-free baking mix
3 teaspoons Homemade Baking Powder
½ teaspoon salt
2 tablespoons ghee
¼ cup almond milk
1 teaspoon powdered vanilla
⅛ cup raw honey
2 teaspoons cinnamon
2 eggs
½ cup raisins
4 tablespoons coconut cream, warmed until liquid
6 tablespoons maguey sap

Instructions:

1. Preheat oven to 400°F.

2. Mix sprouted flour mix, Homemade Baking Powder, and salt together. Add ghee into the mixture to create crumbs.

3. Add almond milk, vanilla powder, cinnamon, and beaten eggs, and mix quickly with a wooden spoon until completely blended.

4. Flour clean countertop and spread your dough. Fold in raisins, and then roll out dough to a 9-inch circle about 3/4" thick.

5. Slice dough evenly into 8–12 pieces, depending upon your size preference. Bake for 15 minutes and cool completely on a cooling rack.

6. While scones are baking, whisk coconut cream and maguey sap in small bowl until smooth to create glaze.

7. Drizzle glaze over your cooled scones.

Tip: place a baking sheet under cooling rack to catch any spilled drizzles.

Variation: to make savory scones, replace the cinnamon, powdered vanilla, and raisins with 3 teaspoons of your favorite Misner Plan seasoning mix or a blend such as herbes de Provence. Serve savory scones with a side dish of olive oil, Lemon Olive Oil, or any of your favorite Misner Plan dressings, instead of the maguey sap glaze.

Sea Salt Caramel Yogurt

Chef Eddie
Serves: 6

I experimented with the idea of crafting a frozen yogurt popsicle, but ended up with this tasty caramel salted yogurt, instead. If you're looking for a replacement for sea-salt caramel ice cream, look no further. The Misner Plan's got you covered!

Ingredients:

1 cup yogurt, goat's or sheep's milk
2 small (or 1 large) vanilla beans
1 tablespoon coconut nectar
1 teaspoon coconut oil
¼ teaspoon cinnamon
Pinch of flaked sea salt (the flakes will dissolve better)
Pinch of Himalayan or other larger crystal sea salt for texture as garnish

Instructions:

1. Scrape the insides of vanilla beans into yogurt and place beans themselves into yogurt to soak for 10–15 minutes.

2. Remove vanilla beans and add coconut nectar, coconut oil, cinnamon, and a pinch of flaked sea salt to the yogurt. Mix well to incorporate all ingredients. Place in the refrigerator to set for approximately 1 hour.

3. When ready to serve, add a pinch of Himalayan or other larger crystal salt to give a crunchy texture.

4. Serve about ¼ cup caramel yogurt in dessert dishes or small ramekins. Serve with Chewy Spiced Ginger Bites.

Tip: for a fluffier dessert, fold in half the meringue topping featured with our Key Lime Pie Bars before refrigerating and stir together gently.

Skillet Corn Bread (Nearly Vegan)

Beth
Serves: 8

I love to eat this skillet corn bread with sprouted black beans, chili, or even with poached eggs. Easy to make and delicious—it satisfies just like Granny's did!

Ingredients:

2 tablespoons grapeseed oil
1 cup gluten-free flour blend
1 cup yellow cornmeal, organic (non-GMO)
1 tablespoon Homemade Baking Powder
1 teaspoon sea salt
1 tablespoon maguey sap
1 cup almond milk
1 large egg white

Instructions:

1. Pour grapeseed oil into a medium cast-iron skillet (about 10 inches in diameter) and place in the oven as it preheats to 375°F.

2. While oil is heating in the skillet, combine flour, cornmeal, Baking Powder, and sea salt in a mixing bowl. Whisk together maguey sap, almond milk, and egg white. Add to the flour mixture and stir just until all ingredients are incorporated. Stir in hot oil from the skillet and then turn batter gently into hot skillet. Return skillet to oven.

3. Bake for 20 minutes or until done in the middle when tested with a toothpick. The top of this corn bread should be golden brown and the sides and bottom should be just a little bit crispy.

Tip: Serve with cooked black beans and onions salted with sea salt as a meal or serve alone as a snack. You can even split open a slice, serving both halves with cooked black beans and onions with a poached egg on each half for a delightful brunch. We like to have some fresh salsa on the side when serving this way.

Part Four

RESOURCES

Thirty

Where to Procure the Obscure

There are some things used in our Misner Plan recipes that might be difficult for you to find at your local market. While many stores are beginning to have a more healthful selection, the Internet is a wonderful place to source the things you may not be able to get at the store.

Here is a list of websites for some of the items we have used in our recipes or have recommended in our book:

Aloe Vera Gel Flakes
http://www.GoodCauseWellness.com

Baking Powder, Aluminum-Free
http://www.bobsredmill.com/baking-powder.html

Bragg's Liquid Aminos
www.bragg.com/products/bragg-liquid-aminos-soy-alternative.html

Broths and Stocks
www.pacificfoods.com/food/broths-stocks.aspx

Buckwheat Groats, Sprouted
www.localharvest.org/organic-sprouted-buckwheat-groats-C22941

Cacao Powder
www.navitasnaturals.com/product/441/Cacao-Powder.htmlCanola Oil

Canola Oil, Non-GMO
www.napavalleynaturals.com

Citrus and Fruit Oils
www.botanicinnovations.com

Coconut Aminos
www.vitacost.com

Coconut Flour
www.bobsredmill.com/organic-coconut-flour.html

Coconut Nectar, Raw
www.coconutsecret.com

Coconut Oil, Expeller Pressed
www.drbronner.com/DBMS/category/COCONUTOIL.html

Coconut Sugar
https://shop.navitasorganics.com/coconut-palm-sugar.html
Cornstarch, Non-GMO
www.swansonvitamins.com/rapunzel-organic-corn-starch-non-gmo-8-oz-pkg

Flour, Einkorn Wheat
https://healthyflour.com

Flours, Sprouted
https://healthyflour.com
www.bluemountainorganics.com/by-type/grains-and-cereals/flours

Gluten-free Flour Blend
https://healthyflour.com

Grains, Sprouted
www.truroots.com

Grapeseed Oil
www.napavalleynaturals.com

Honey, Healing Manuka, Raw
www.thesynergycompany.com

Maguey Sweet Sap Syrup
www.amazon.com/Organic-Maguey-Sweet-Syrup-23-65/dp/B008FJYDG0

Nuts and Seeds, Sprouted
www.bluemountainorganics.com/by-type/seeds-and-nuts/sprouted-nuts-seeds

Olive Oil
www.bragg.com/products/bragg-organic-extra-virgin-olive-oil.html
www.conolivos.com

Pastas, Gluten-Free
www.jovialfoods.com

Raisins, Golden/Sultana
www.naturalhealinghouse.com

Red Palm Fruit Oil
store.nutiva.com/red-palm-oil

Seaweed
www.seaveg.com

Seeds, Sprouted
https://www.goraw.com/shop/sprouted-seeds/

Spices
www.simplyorganic.com

Stevia, Whole-Leaf
www.bulkapothecary.com

Supplements
Premier Research Laboratories
www.pureformulas.com

Tea seed Oil
www.aretteorganic.com/Arette-Tea-Oil-Shop.html

Thrive Market
https://thrivemarket.com

Tulsi Teas
www.organicindiausa.com/tulsi-tea

Vanilla, Powdered
http://www.sunfood.com/herbs-teas-spices/vanilla-bean-powder.html

White Vinegar, Non-GMO
www.spectrumorganics.com/spectrum-naturals/white-vinegar-org-distilled

Epilogue

Ivan
with Dr. Miguel Espinoza

After all our hard work and diligence, imagine our dismay when my PSA count started becoming elevated once again in May of 2016. Remembering that my doctors had told me to watch my numbers carefully, because prostate cancer is one of the cancers that can often reoccur, I was diligent to go for regular testing. Three years after hearing my treating physician in California say, "You are in remission," my new urologist in Texas told me. "I want to do an MRI to see what's going on," he added. My PSA count had risen to over 13.

The scan revealed three tiny lesions. I knew then there was going to be more to my story.

I'm very happy to begin this epilogue by telling you that just last week my treating urologist told me after conducting an exam, "Your prostate feels fine." He went on to tell me to come back in six months for another scan and to keep an eye on the PSA level, which is 0.3 (or nearly zero) as of today.

This final chapter of our book will address a crucial healing phase of my journey. Remember that I said from the outset I believe Western medicine may need to be part of my healing process. But when and where natural, alternative healthcare can work to my advantage, I plan to take that approach. It definitely may not be for everyone, and it may ultimately not be all I use, but it has not let me down yet!

After several consultations with my urologist, his conclusion was that he wanted to do an ultrasound-guided biopsy to, as he put it, "be sure of the molecular composition of the tissue." At this point, he did not feel HIFU would be an appropriate treatment for the lesions. He was leaning toward a recommendation of either radiation or a radical prostatectomy. He did not seem able to comprehend that I was not scared, which gave me the confidence to choose a slower, less invasive and less damaging form of effective treatment. When a radical prostatectomy would have completely resolved my experience with cancer, he did not understand why I might not elect to have him go in and just cut out my prostate gland at this early stage or bombard it with nuclear medicine's finest photon beams.

The risks still seemed to me to be highly undesirable, and there was no evidence that any of the lesions were on the verge of escaping the capsule.

Wanting to be sure that the recommendation he was leaning toward was consistent with best medical practices, I opted to get a second opinion. The doctor I consulted next was in agreement with him, and enlightened me that most of the side effects of both targeted radiation and radical prostatectomy were reversible in most of his patients' cases. While that thought was comforting, when he explained some of the ways his patients' bodies adjust to intimacy when there is no prostate gland, I had even more reason to really get serious about whatever additional alternative plan I wanted to try right now before getting on THAT path!

Beth and I started looking into alternative healthcare centers in the United States where I might go for several weeks to completely detox and get on some targeted therapies for my condition, such as juicing or other natural modalities. While we considered what was available, Beth researched the use of pancreatic enzymes in conjunction with traditional cancer treatment, and I started using pancreatic enzymes between meals. We followed up on an earlier recommendation from Dr. Kellas to include hedge apples in my diet. I tightened up my meal plan and got back on Phase 2, eliminating all fruits; natural sweeteners; red meats, including wild meats and lamb; and all dairy, including goat's milk yogurt and cheeses.

Then one of our BNI members in Southern California messaged Beth with a referral to a medical doctor practicing just south of the US border near San Diego, Dr. Isai Castillo at Clínica CIPAG. We had a few e-mail exchanges with Dr. Castillo and a couple of phone calls to learn more about his approach.

He told us that if I were to come to his medical center, he would conduct a thorough physical examination and do extensive lab work to get the readings from the major body systems, such as the immune, endocrine, and renal systems in order to evaluate my overall health, and he might wish to refer me to some other specialists for additional examinations, X-rays, and other scans.

He also mentioned that he sometimes uses chemotherapy with his cancer patients, and sometimes recommends surgery if he believes it to be helpful. He, of course, puts his patients on targeted nutritional supplementation and a wide variety of complementary treatments, such as IV therapy, hyperbaric chamber, dietary recommendations, and herbal preparations as indicated by their conditions.

Pleased with what we learned and encouraged by the fact that Dr. Castillo seemed to have one foot in Western medicine and the other in alternative therapies, we made plans to travel to Baja California to see how his twenty-one-day protocol would affect my condition. CIPAG is a medical center, not a retreat/treatment facility. Although his medical center has a few suites on the top floors of the building, most of his patients stay either in the San Diego area, coming to his clinic for their daily treatments, or they stay locally in Tijuana. We opted for the latter.

I have to tell you that we were very pleased with the treatment I received. Dr. Castillo has a team of doctors working with him and a nursing staff who are competent and caring. My first day there was full with the intake procedure, giving my health history to Dr. Miguel Espinoza, having a complete physical examination, blood work, and another PSA test. The treatment started the same day.

I have asked Dr. Espinoza to join me in writing this chapter:

(Dr. Miguel Espinoza) When I evaluated Ivan, I was encouraged to learn that he had gone into remission once before. In my experience, it is easier to get positive results quickly when that has been the case, especially if the malignancy is still contained within the prostate gland.

To reduce inflammation in Ivan's body and boost his immune system, I recommended that he start with IV therapy (vitamin C, sodium bicarbonate, glutathione, DMSO chelation, and B-17/Laetrile), take effervescent vitamin C tablets three times per day, drink guanabana (also known as sour sop or graviola) tea twenty minutes before eating each meal, and drink my fresh Baja Healing Juice.

To make Baja Healing Juice, process together in a VitaMix: a beet, a carrot, two pieces of broccoli, a medium bell pepper, a celery stalk, three slices of onion, a radish, a garlic clove, and half a glass of spring water. Blend until completely smooth. Pour into a large glass through a sieve, then add the juice of one lemon to the liquid.

While conducting Ivan's physical exam, I noticed that he has pretty bad sinus problems. I referred him to an ear, nose, throat specialist whom he was able to see the next day.

I also recommended that he begin going into the hyperbaric chamber daily after having a chest X-ray to be sure there was no lung condition that would contraindicate that therapy. We requested a driver associated with the radiology clinic to take him to get the X-ray, which I was able to evaluate the very same day.

Ivan saw Dr. Castillo for his review and additional recommendations on the third day. Ivan's lungs looked great, and he was cleared for the oxygen therapy. We had Ivan's current PSA by this time, which had dropped from 13 to 7.12 since May. Probably the things Ivan and Beth had started to do at home (starting on Phase 2, taking the pancreatic enzymes, and adding hedge apples to Ivan's diet) were moving things in the right direction.

I also prescribed hormone-blocking medication for him. There would be some side effects to this hormone blocker, so I prescribed another medication to help offset them. The hormone blocker works to suppress testosterone levels so the rest of the treatments can have maximum impact on supporting the body while it sets about reducing inflammation in the prostate gland. The medication prescribed has been medically proven to shrink prostate cancer lesions. Ironically, it is not distributed in America. One doctor asked the pharmaceutical company about why it is not available there and was told, "It's so cheap that there is no money in using it." It is not banned, but it simply is not available, so it is not prescribed by doctors in the United States.

What Ivan was about to do here with us was targeted to put his body's healing processes into overdrive.

I recommended that he stayed in the Misner Plan's Phase 2 and that he add an herbal tonic. I also prescribed live cell injections which have been shown to support the immune system. The live bovine immune cells help the body heal other cellular damage so one's own immune cells can focus on taking care of any other inflammation, specifically for Ivan in the prostate gland.

(Ivan) Once he ordered all these elements of the protocol, Dr. Espinoza said my PSA level would be checked again at the end of the second week I was doing their treatments.

I had a fairly uncomfortable reaction to the IV therapy. I have quite small veins, and it is difficult for most nurses to insert an IV catheter. As a result, the various infusions tend to burn as they are being delivered, and they go in very slowly. Most people at the clinic finished their infusions within about forty-five minutes. Mine took about twice as long and were very uncomfortable.

Dr. Espinoza asked me to consider having either a port or a central line catheter put in to make the twenty-one-day treatment protocol more comfortable for me. Since a port is permanent and would not be removed at the end of the twenty-one days, I opted for the central line. I was told I would need to go to a surgical center to have the surgeon associated with Clínica CIPAG insert the central line. My appointment was made for first thing the next morning.

A private driver picked us up at our hotel. By the way, the hotel we stayed in has an entire floor set up as a recovery wing for guests healing from various procedures ranging from cosmetic surgery to minor cancer surgeries, complete with nursing staff, doctor visits, movies on demand, and room service! We learned that more than eighty of the current hotel guests were in Mexico for "medical tourism," getting various types of medical treatment.

We were driven to a private hospital. Amazing. This was something I have never experienced; that's for sure. The surgeon told me what he needed to do to insert the central line catheter, a procedure that would only take about eight to ten minutes, during which time would be lightly sedated for my comfort.

After waiting in my private room for over thirty minutes, Beth began to grow worried. When the orderly poked his head in to let her know what was going on, she learned that my procedure was more complicated than anticipated. But eventually the procedure was successfully completed, and I left quite sore, but ready for the IV treatments. Having the central line sure made everything easier, more comfortable, and quicker. I also had both hands free now, so I was able to continue writing, keep up with my e-mails, and work during the three weeks I was getting my treatment.

What Beth did not expect was how she would react to seeing me with tubes coming out of my body and all the bruising on my chest from the surgeon's difficulties in inserting the line. Always my rock, she shared with me later that she felt really shaken up during that time. She became even more concerned and quite anxious, hovering over me for every little thing. Truth be told, I kind of liked it! She told me later that the full realization that I had relapsed had all come down on her at that point.

Her support during the treatment was really wonderful. She helped me keep track of the supplement schedule, made the IV treatments more efficient by ordering our lunch so I could eat while having the treatments, and even found an organic restaurant right across the street from our hotel for healthy Misner Plan breakfasts and dinners. I can honestly say that my three weeks there was much more manageable because of her presence and active participation. There were other couples there, and it was apparent that the patients with support were able to cope far better because of their partner's attentiveness. I could not imagine going through this process all alone.

I was not looking forward to the recommended hyperbaric medicine, but Dr. Espinoza clarified the benefits to me of breathing oxygen under pressure, and I became convinced it would be helpful. We've asked Dr. Espinoza to share his explanation with you:

(Dr. Miguel Espinoza) First of all, there are two things to know about cancer: cancer loves sugar, and cancer hates oxygen. If cancer loves sugar, don't feed the body "bad" sugar (processed, easily converted to glucose). If cancer hates oxygen, give the body oxygen. There are some cancers, such as melanoma, where this is not the case, but I will talk about that in a moment.

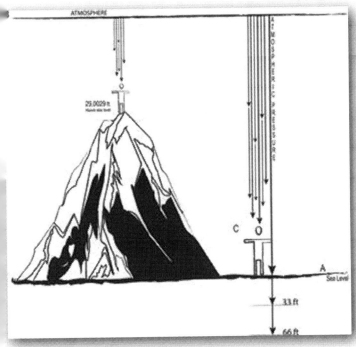

Dr. Espinoza went through this explanation with a sheet of white paper between us, drawing a diagram upside down (fig. 1), so we could see the elements of his description.

I am drawing a line right here at sea level (A), and a line right here, which represents the atmosphere (B). And I'm drawing a line to represent you standing at sea level (C).

We know that there is air exerting pressure on your body. This pressure is called...?

Beth and I both replied, "Atmospheric pressure."

Atmospheric pressure is considered to be one atmosphere at sea level (approximately 14.7 psi), and varies, depending on how far above sea level you are. For example, if you are on top of Mount Everest, which is located at 29,029 feet above sea level, the atmospheric pressure is going to be less. Why? Because you have less quantity of air exerting pressure on your body. The atmospheric pressure is going to be 0.4, OK?

Beth and I nodded in understanding.

Now, climbers have to wear oxygen masks when they climb. You're probably going to ask me why. A lot of my patients think it is because there is a lack of oxygen on top of Mount Everest. (*He indicated the summit by drawing a bold arrow.*) No, it's not. It's because of the lack of pressure.

A lack of pressure does not let the lungs expand enough to absorb an adequate amount of oxygen. So basically, the less pressure being exerted on your body, the less your body is going to be receiving adequate amounts of oxygen, OK?

We again shook our heads in agreement.

So, if up here at the summit I have less pressure, and down here at sea level I have more pressure, how can I get even *more* pressure? Well, by going under sea level.

For every thirty-three feet we go under sea level, we're going to add one atmosphere more. For example, if we're thirty-three feet below sea level, we're going to be having a total of two atmospheres: one for the pressure of air and one for the pressure of water under sea level. How about if we go sixty-six feet under sea level? We're going to have a total of three on the body: one for the air and two for the underwater pressure.

And why is there such a huge difference with only thirty-three and sixty-six feet under sea level compared to nearly thirty thousand feet above sea level for the summit of Mount Everest? Simply, the density of water is far greater than air.

In the hyperbaric chamber, we can increase the air pressure to match the pressure of being thirty-three feet under sea level and under that amount of water pressure to give the patients two atmospheres of pressure on their body. It simulates the underwater pressure.

When we put you in the chamber and increase the air pressure, we give you a special mask like a pilot's mask. Like *Top Gun*! We give you 100 percent oxygen plus more pressure to increase the oxygen levels in your body. By doing this, we give you about forty times more oxygen than what you are going to have at sea level. This percentage varies by patient, since everybody is different, but that's a general amount of increased oxygenation.

If you have forty times more oxygen, and cancer does not like oxygen, cancer is not going to be able to thrive. There is a theory that says higher oxygen levels create more blood vessels in the body, and that by creating more blood vessels you have more cancer activity. This is why we screen our patients carefully so we are sure not to use it on melanoma for which this is true, but that doesn't happen with the type of cancer Ivan was diagnosed with: adenocarcinoma.

Before going into the hyperbaric chamber, we ask every patient to see a hyperbaric medicine specialist so we are sure the patient is a good candidate for this protocol. If the hyperbaric medicine specialist says, "No, this is not a good candidate for the hyperbaric chamber," we won't put that patient in for hyperbaric medicine.

Hyperbaric medicine is considered anything above 1.4 atmospheres. Everything below that level is not hyperbaric medicine.

At this point, Beth asked if it is true that lab techs who work with cancer cells in petri dishes stop cancer from multiplying when they go home at night by inserting an oxygen tube into the dish. Dr. Espinoza confirmed that is correct. Research scientists know how to stop cancer cells from multiplying: give them more oxygen.

When I learned I was going to be in a small, enclosed chamber for at least an hour each day, wearing a *Top Gun* mask, potentially in close contact with five strangers, without the ability to have my reading glasses to even read for that hour, I was not excited. I can honestly tell you that I did not consider the networking opportunities at the time. But what I experienced was a bit different. I even grew to sort of enjoy the therapy, and I have missed it after coming back home.

There were small windows in the chamber that gave it a miniature submarine look. There was also a TV in the chamber, so the therapist let me pick a movie to watch during my session. Fortunately, I was able to watch the first half of the movie on day one, and then the second half of the movie on day two. And often, because I chose to start my day with the hyperbaric therapy and most of the patients chose to go straight to the IV therapy, I was alone or with only one or two others, so the chamber did not feel quite as small.

I discovered something quite comfortable very early in my sessions. Whenever my body was in the pressurized chamber for a certain length of time, my muscles relaxed, and I could get a really nice spinal release when I gently stretched my neck and back. It was like seeing a full-spine chiropractor every day. It turned out that one of the things I was least looking forward to ended up being one of the most relaxing and restful parts of the treatment process.

Remember that Dr. Espinoza referred me to an ear, nose, and throat specialist? Well, it was a good thing my bride is fluent in Spanish for that visit, for sure. He did not speak English.

She served as the translator as he got my health history and heard about my sinus problems, problems I have had for many years.

He explained that there was a lot of inflammation in my nasal passages: enough that it was inhibiting my body's ability to bring in high enough levels of oxygen when I breathe, especially at night. Just as hyperbaric medicine assists the body with obtaining higher levels of oxygen, having decreased inflammation in the nasal pathways could also help with my oxygen level. He recommended cauterizing my nasal passages or prescribing a special inhaler to assist with reducing the inflammation. When he explained through Beth that I would likely have to repeat the cauterization in order to find relief, I opted for the inhaler.

I was really holding on to hope that my next blood test result would show the treatments were lowering my PSA levels. I was doing so many things to support my body's healing processes. With great anticipation, I had a blood draw to check where things were midway through my second week of treatment. The results came in a couple of days later.

By the end of that second week, my PSA level was down from 7.12 to 3.81. I was elated. This result was what I was hoping for. Dr. Espinoza told me that everything we were doing was turning down the heat, so to speak, which was helping my body lower the levels of inflammation and reducing size of the likely malignant lesions. I was really pleased. I knew the final PSA test at Clínca CIPAG would probably be lower still, but what I did not know was how the results from their lab would compare with the testing and results from my lab at home.

I had the final blood draw at CIPAG a few of days before concluding my twenty-one-day treatment. The results would be in on my last day, I was told. Beth and I both nearly held our breath, waiting to hear where things stood.

On the day before my last day, Dr. Espinoza easily removed the central line catheter. It had been a long three weeks, and we were ready to return home to Texas. Having the central line out heightened our anticipation of getting that last PSA reading and then flying home.

On the last day, we both looked at each other in stunned silence as the final result came in: 2.1. My PSA went from 7.12 to 2.1 in just twenty-one days. When I looked back to the test result at the height of my relapse, I realized the drop was really from just above 13 over a period of five months. Beth and I were both really encouraged.

We prepared to leave Clínica CIPAG by getting all the recommended supplements and medications together to return home for the next three months before coming back for a ten-day follow-up. Dr. Castillo sent me home with a prescription for the supplements *and* the medications to have with me for travel. There was no problem crossing the border, since none of the items prescribed by the medical center are actually banned or prohibited in the United States.

As soon as we returned home, I went directly to my lab in Austin and had another PSA test performed so that I could compare the results from my usual lab with the lab at Clínica CIPAG. Absolutely gobsmacked, we learned that my PSA reading was now 1.4. Dr. Castillo had told me at the very first appointment I had with him that his goal was to see my PSA drop to nearly zero. At the time, I thought, "It's good to have goals." OK, to be honest, I might have actually even said this later to Beth.

What was actually happening was getting very close to his near-zero goal.

Upon settling into our new routine at home, Beth learned how to give me B17 shots, which were recommended three times per week. Since I came home with a new supplement schedule, I had to adjust to taking various micronutrients on a very choreographed timeline. With my busy lifestyle and travel schedule, this has not been easy to do. The hormone blocker makes me extremely nauseous, and the hormonal changes have also been hard to adjust to, but I keep telling myself that it is all temporary. Dr. Castillo told me that as my PSA moved closer to zero, he would reduce the dose, so that would help reduce the impact of the side effects.

The week before my return to Clínica CIPAG for the recommended ten-day, follow-up treatment, I had another PSA test result come in. This time I went public with my results. The current reading, as of the close of this epilogue, is 0.3. Yes, you read that correctly: very nearly zero.

I also took my results and current condition back to my treating urologist in Austin. When he saw my most recent PSA score, his first question was, "Who have you seen since you last saw me?" He went on to listen as I shared everything I had done. Then I asked him what he thought about the results from it all. He said bluntly, "You already know my bias. I've explained it about ten times. I'm not going to go over it again with you folks." Beth thought he was firing me as a patient!

But after doing a physical exam of my prostate, he said, "Your prostate feels fine."

"My prostate feels fine?" I repeated with a question in my voice, wondering about the bulge he had detected previously.

A bit more tersely he repeated, "Your prostate feels fine. I'd like to see you back in about six months for another MRI scan. Keep an eye on your PSA in the meantime."

I'm grateful that he did not fire me, because I do want him on my team.

You may be reading this, wondering if I paid a fortune to go to a specialized medical center in Mexico, out-of-pocket, not covered by my medical insurance because of how far out of the paradigm of our traditional Western medical establishment this approach is. I can tell you this: Dr. Castillo's approach is not the same as the resort-like retreats you may have read about on the beach in Baja California. His modalities are both alternative and medical. I like that combination. And I will tell you this, I paid about one-third of what the typical twenty-one-day retreats charge, and there was no companion fee for my bride to tag along.

While it's true that my medical insurance is not going to cover a single penny of what Dr. Castillo prescribed, including medical X-rays, IVs, prescriptions, etc., I am confident that I made the right choice for me. The type of treatment one chooses when faced with a serious diagnosis is very personal. My thinking is that I need all the information I can get regarding the different approaches toward healing.

Even now, knowing what I do about so-called alternative healthcare, I still want to consult traditional Western medicine practitioners. It's important to see all sides of an issue. Medical doctors have training that gives them a particular perspective. I believe it's important to consider that perspective. And I don't have to agree with doctors to want them on my team. Hearing all sides is important to make an informed decision.

I remain the captain of my ship, and I will make decisions that work best for my health. I recommend that others get all the information they can, even if it means considering positions they disagree with, so they can make an informed decision for themselves. I do not tell my story to persuade you to avoid "standard" medical procedures or to encourage you do something you may not have confidence in. I tell my story simply to illustrate that there may be alternatives to how medical issues can be approached and with hope that you will make changes you know you need to make even when not diagnosed with something serious in order to have a long, healthy, productive life. If my story helps you to make preventive changes in your own kitchen regarding how you nourish your body and to begin avoiding chemicals in what you eat that may increase inflammation in your body, then I will be very glad.

In the case of my specific diagnosis, I was presented with three paths. The very *first* path offered to me was the nuclear option: radiation. The second path I was offered was radical: complete prostatectomy. The third path offered to me was akin to chemical warfare: traditional chemotherapy.

The path I chose was one I had to seek out. It was a path that followed the trail of the probable cause of my condition: inflammation. And it was a nonviolent path. I am not sure why I came out of remission and experienced a reoccurrence of prostate cancer, but I am sure that the path I chose led me to today, when Dr. Espinoza gratefully said the words I have been waiting to hear again: "You are in complete remission now. Enjoy your life!"

Acknowledgments

From Ivan and Beth Misner: We would not have had such a positive outcome in Ivan's experience without the support and input from several key players on Ivan's medical team. Many, many heartfelt thanks go to Drs. Bill Kellas, Mark LaBeau, Edward Davis, Kevin Kelly, Daniel Amen, Mohammad Nikkhah, Bill Nelson (also a Misner Plan advisory-board member), Isai Castillo, and Miguel Espinoza, who worked with both of us personally. Further input from authors, including Drs. Mark Sholz, Mark Hyman, William Li, Bernie Siegel, and T. Colin Campbell, helped us stay on the right path for healing. We are indebted to you, too.

We would also like to acknowledge the support of our family, especially our children, Ashley, Cassandra, and Trey. Although you may have not been sure Dad was doing the right thing, you were great about reserving judgment until you began to see results. We both love you so much and are extremely grateful that we have many healthy years ahead of us together as a family!

We are grateful to Eric Edmeades (a Misner Plan advisory-board member), who suggested that we create the Misner Plan as a way to share what we have experienced and learned through this experience. Thanks so much for planting seeds that have borne so much fruit.

To our other two Misner Plan advisory-board members, Dr. Lise Janelle and Dr. Fabrizio Mancini, thank you for your support, input, and constant encouragement. You have been wonderful.

Acknowledgments

Special thanks go to Patty Aubery, president of Jack Canfield Inc., your support of our work and this book project has encouraged us greatly.

Tanja Schneider, your work on the recipes was immensely helpful. Thank you for taking time to work with us tirelessly to catalog and chart our recipes to get things organized.

And to our coauthor and collaborator on the book, Chef Eddie Esposito—wow, you rock. Your delicious recipes have helped us stay completely engaged with our own plan. We are certain that many people will benefit by recapturing their health and being able to stay engaged with the Misner Plan because of your creativity in the kitchen. Thank you!

From Chef Eddie Esposito: When it comes to cooking and my culinary journey, there are a few people who were instrumental in my journey of traveling the world and cooking for celebrities. The most influential individuals have been Drago and Klara Cvitanovich of Drago's restaurant in New Orleans. Immigrants to the United States from communist Yugoslavia, Drago and Klara took me in as a sixteen-year-old and gave me my first taste of the restaurant business, cooking, and world travel—things that still drive me today. I also credit you both with teaching me the most important things in life—God; family; and a tireless, enthusiastic work ethic.

I thank my good friend Larry Thibodeaux, who gave me my first job cooking in the air. You still push me to try new things, sending me pictures from all over the world of foods you encounter so we can have an interesting dinner during the too-few times we seem to be able to get together.

My family and my coauthors are all amazing. My wife, Heather, was a good palate! You were such a great hostess for me and our various guests during our testing weekends. Beth, you brought the vision and the guidance to complete this task. You are a brilliant, powerful, and inspiring woman. Ivan, how can I ever thank you enough for your courage and inspiration in sharing this personal journey with all of us? When I think about what it took for you to do what you have done, I am humbled and amazed.

I thank all of you and look forward to seeing you and your families in good health.

About the Authors

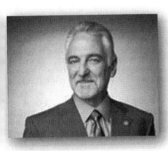

Dr. Ivan Misner is the founder and chief visionary officer of BNI (Business Network Int'l.). He is a *New York Times* best-selling author, entrepreneur, and the cofounder of the BNI Foundation and Asentiv. His drive and initiative have touched many people all over the globe. His recent experience with prostate cancer has also had an impact not only in his BNI organization but also with friends and family. Ivan's Givers Gain attitude has allowed him to share openly about his path and choices regarding comprehensive health care to move into wellness. Websites: www.IvanMisner.com and www.MisnerPlan.com.

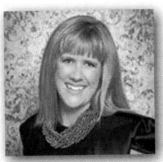

Beth Misner is the corporate vice chair emeritus of BNI; the cofounder of the BNI Foundation; and founder of the Journey Center in Claremont, California. She is a certified chiropractic assistant, certified sports nutritionist, black belt in karate, tai chi chuan and qigong instructor, ordained minister, and meditation leader. When Ivan was diagnosed in 2012 with prostate cancer, she drew from all her expertise relating to the mind, body, and spirit connection to partner with him on a journey into recovered health. Websites: www.BethMisner.com and www.MisnerPlan.com.

About the Authors

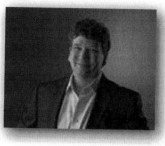

Eddie Esposito is cofounder and vice president of Asentiv and a certified business and life coach. He was a restaurateur whose restaurant was featured in the culinary magazine *Bon Appétit*. He owned and operated one of the top-ten private-aircraft catering companies in the world, where he was the corporate jet chef for President Jimmy Carter, President George H. W. Bush, President Bill Clinton, President George W. Bush, and First Lady Michelle Obama, as well as a bevy of movie stars. He combines his love of the culinary arts with his current corporate role, helping Asentiv franchise owners and clients worldwide experience a spectacular life that includes the enjoyment of wonderfully delicious foods. His passion for Cajun/Creole New Orleans cuisine makes its way into just about every dish he creates.

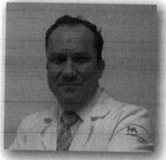

Dr. Miguel Angel Espinoza holds a medical degree as a physician surgeon from Universidad Xochicalco (CEUX), Mexico; a naturopathy degree from Guatemala University; and a master's degree in public health and nutrition from Loma Linda University in California, USA. In addition, Dr. Espinoza is a board-certified diplomate in both emergency medicine from Universidad Nacional Autónoma de México (UNAM) and undersea and hyperbaric medicine from Instituto Politécnico Nacional (IPN), Mexico. He currently practices medicine at Clínica CIPAG in Tijuana, Baja California, Mexico.

Follow us on Facebook: https://www.facebook.com/MisnerPlan

Subject Index

Recipe Index

Recipe Index

Made in the USA
San Bernardino, CA
21 October 2017